Keto Soups Cookbook

*100 Fat Burning & Delicious Soups, Stews, Broths
& Bread Asian for Busy People on Keto Diet*

Lara Fisch

The trademarks that are used are without any consent, and the publication of the trademark is without permission or backing by the trademark owner. All trademarks and brands within this book are for clarifying purposes only and are the owned by the owners themselves, not affiliated with this document.

Table of contents

Introduction

With mortality risk as high as 2.9 million annually, obesity continues to be a significant global health risk amid continuous advancements in the medical field. The bulk of cardiovascular disorders such as diabetes, asthma, and heart problems are primarily attributed to obesity, which is generally a result of destructive eating patterns and unhealthy lifestyles. Appropriately formulated weight loss diet medications can work to some degree to manage the obesity crisis. A super-low-carbohydrate and the high-fat keto diet is one diet plan that proves to be super-efficient for rapid weight loss.

Increased-fats, modest-proteins, and quite-low-carbohydrates are mainly part of a ketogenic diet. About 56% to 61% fat, 31 percent to 36 percent protein and 6 percent to 11 percent carbohydrates are classified into dietary macro and micronutrients. Primarily, carbohydrates amount to 20–40g a day in a 1900kcal regular diet.

The ketogenic diet was first used by Russel Wilder to cure epilepsy. He also invented the word "ketogenic diet." The keto diet maintained a role as a preventive diet for childhood epilepsy in the medical community for almost a decade. It was commonly used before its popularity ended with the advent of antiepileptic drugs. The revival of the ketogenic diet as a formula for accelerated weight loss is a relatively recent phenomenon that, at least in the short term, has proved to be very successful.

A relatively low-carbohydrates, high-fat diet that has specific links to the Atkins and low-carbohydrates diets is the ketogenic diet. It requires significantly lowering and replacing the intake of carbohydrates with fat. This carbohydrate reduction places the body in a metabolic condition called ketosis. One's body gets incredibly good at consuming fat for energy as this occurs. It also converts fat into liver ketone bodies, which can provide the brain with energy.

This book "Keto Soups Cookbook" is a complete guide about the ketogenic diet and its benefits along with more than 100 recipes of soups and vegetarian foods that can make you feel warm and comfortable in winter. Chapter 1 and 2 are about basic introduction of the ketogenic diet, its benefits, risks, foods to eat and food to avoid, shopping list and making keto diet your lifestyle. Chapter 3 and 4 will provide you with tasty soup recipes around the world. Chapter 5 is all about winter comfort foods and spicy, delicious dishes. Chapter 6 is a vegetarian section with breakfast, lunch and dinner recipes. Thus, Start reading the book and learn a lot of new and exciting things about the ketogenic diet and keto-friendly recipes.

Chapter 1: Understanding Ketogenic Diet and Benefits

The ketogenic diet is mainly around the idea that you should pressure the body to consume fat for food by draining the body from carbohydrates, which are its primary source of nutrition, thereby optimizing fat loss. Keto, which means the low-carb, high-fat ketogenic diet, tends to be the most recent buzzword to enter the diet community. So what exactly is a ketogenic diet, and are you right about the weight reduction program? Before you decide to get over your eating behavior and attitudes, let us take a closer look.

1.1 How Ketogenic Diet Works

The ketogenic weight loss diet is founded on the notion that maximum fat loss can be accomplished by driving the body into ketosis. Ketosis is a natural metabolic mechanism that happens when there are inadequate glucose reserves for energy in the body. Once these reserves are drained, instead of carbohydrates, the body returns to consume the stored fat for energy. Acids called ketones, which form up in the body and can be used for energy, are generated by this process.

1.2 Types of Ketogenic Diet

Different types of ketogenic diet are available. Most people who adopt a ketogenic diet assume the so-called traditional ketogenic diet schedule, which contains around 10 % of total carbohydrate calories. Cyclic ketogenic diets, also recognized as carb cycling, and targeted ketogenic diets, which allow for changes in carbohydrate consumption during exercise, are the other types of ketogenic diets. Typically, these improvements are undertaken by athletes who wish to use the ketogenic diet to increase strength and recovery and not by people primarily focusing on weight loss.

But broadly speaking, you can try to eat less than 10% of the total carbohydrate calorie a day because you intend to adopt a ketogenic diet. 15 to 20 percent protein and 70 to 75 per cent fat should come from the leftover calories. That means no upwards of 200 of your calories (or 60 gram) should come from carbohydrates if you adopt a regular 2,000-calorie diet, whereas 500 to 650 calories should come from proteins and 1,300 to 1,500 from fat.

1.3 Health Benefits of Ketogenic Diet

Related to most low-carb and greater-fat diets, the advantages of a ketogenic diet are similar, but it tends to be more efficient than moderate low-carb diets. Thoughts of keto as an amazingly-charged, low-carb diet, enhancing the advantages. It can also, however, raise the risk of side effects a little.

Weight Loss

For weight loss, converting the body into a fat-burning device may be helpful. Fat burning is dramatically improved, while sugar levels decrease significantly, the fat-store hormone which tends to make it much easier for body fat reduction to occur, without appetite.

About forty high-quality clinical trials indicate that low-carbohydrate and ketogenic diets lead to more successful weight loss relative to other diets.

Reverse Type 2 Diabetes

Studies suggest that a ketogenic diet is excellent for the treatment of type 2 diabetes, often sometimes resulting in remission of the disease. It makes common sense because keto lowers the amount of blood sugar, decreases the need for medicine, and decreases the possible detrimental influence of elevated levels of insulin. Since a keto diet will reverse current type 2 diabetes, as well as cure pre-diabetes, it is likely to be successful in combating it. In the best-case situation, it can be increased to such a degree that blood glucose falls to usual without long-term treatment.

Appetite Control

You would achieve greater control of the appetite on a keto diet. The dramatically declining feelings of hunger is a very normal occurrence, and research shows it. This typically makes it possible to eat very little and lose excess weight. It also makes it much easier to fast intermittently, something that will boost attempts to cure type two diabetes and accelerate weight loss, despite the effects of just keto. Additionally, by not trying to eat all the time, you might save money and time. On a keto diet, many people have the urge to feed twice a day, and others only feed once a day.

Calm your Stomach

A keto diet can lead to a calmer abdomen, less air, less constipation and less pain, also leading to changes in the symptoms of IBS. This is the greatest asset for certain persons, and it also only takes a day or two to feel it.

Mental Performance and Energy

For improved mental performance, certain persons explicitly use ketogenic diets. It is also normal for individuals to feel an increase in energy when ketosis is activated. On keto, there is no need for dietary carbs in mind. It is driven by ketones 24/7 along with a lower amount of liver-synthesized glucose. There is no requirement for carbs in the diet.

Therefore, ketosis helps in a constant supply of fuel (ketones) to the brain, thereby preventing complications with significant fluctuations of blood sugar. This will sometimes result in better attention and concentration, with improved mental comprehension, and mental fogginess resolution.

Epilepsy

A proven and frequently successful medicinal treatment for epilepsy that was first used in the 19th century is the ketogenic diet. It has historically been used mainly for youth, but adults have also learned from it in recent times. Using a ketosis epilepsy diet can enable some individuals to take less or no antiepileptic drugs at all, while probably staying seizure-free. This can decrease the side effects of drugs and thus improve mental performance.

Physical Endurance

In principle, ketogenic diets will improve your physical stamina by enhancing your access to the large quantities of energy in your stored fat. The body's stock of processed carbohydrates survives only for a few hours or less of vigorous exercise. Yet your fat reserves hold enough energy to last for weeks theoretically. Beyond this impact, the decrease in the amount of body fat that can be obtained on a keto diet is another possible advantage. In a variety of athletic events, like endurance athletics, this decrease in body fat weight is highly beneficial.

1.4 Risks for Ketogenic Diet and How to Minimize?

It is important to know what research says and how it will impact your health before you give this diet strategy a shot. Indeed, you will want to be mindful of the possible risks of keto diets.

Fatigue and Keto Flu

The "keto flu" is among the most frequent side effects of initiating the ketogenic diet. This concept explains the often painful, inflammation-inducing symptoms as the body transitions to a low-carbohydrate food from a high-carbohydrate diet. The body's accumulated glucose starts to be exhausted during the keto flu, and the brain continues to respond to the development and use of ketones as energy. Keto flu symptoms include fever, nausea, dizziness, difficulty sleeping, cramps, palpitations, and diarrhoea. Usually, these side effects diminish and ultimately disappear after about two weeks. But actually, try moving slowly into a ketogenic diet rather than trying to change your dietary habits to minimize the consequences of any pain. Through decreasing your carbohydrate consumption steadily, whilst growing your dietary fat intake progressively over time, you will transition with less of a detrimental effect and possibly avoid keto flu.

Constipation

It may contribute to its collection of gastrointestinal side effects by eliminating several grains and fruits with such a strong focus on fats. Constipation and diarrhoea with Keto are not rare. If not handled well, you cannot get enough fibre, which may lead to constipation, with much of your carbs originating from fibre-rich veggies.

Nutritional Deficiency

Sometimes, ketogenic diets are deficient in potassium, calcium, vitamin D, magnesium, and folic acid, which can lead to nutritional deficits over time if the diet is not adequately prepared.

Prevention from Side Effects

Start transforming the meal schedule gradually to avoid side effects, such as keto flu. Begin by learning how much carbohydrates you take in the majority of days. Then start reducing your consumption of carbohydrates steadily throughout a couple of weeks while steadily increasing your dietary fat consumption to maintain your calories the same. To guarantee that this approach works well for you and your fitness priorities, you can also make sure to get advice from a specialist. See a nutritionist and adjust the diet to suit your long-term needs.

The strategy could also be challenging to stick to in the long term because of the heavy carb limits and exclusion of foods such as grains. It can lead to weight spinning or yo-yo dieting to start the diet, give it up, and try it again, in turn making it difficult to lose weight overall. Be sure to contact the healthcare provider and, if possible, a licensed nutritionist to ensure that you fulfil the dietary requirements with the menu if you are willing to follow the keto diet. Consulting with a trainer will help you decide whether you can make improvements or if you would be better off quitting the diet.

1.5 Turning Ketogenic Diet into your Lifestyle

To follow a diet that significantly reduces carbs, it is important to track your food choices closely to ensure that you satisfy your nutritional needs. Consulting a certified dietitian, without raising the chance of complications or harmful side effects, will guarantee that you safely practice this diet. It is important to note that the purpose of any dietary adjustment is to encourage a healthier lifestyle, so make sure you choose a long-term meal schedule that you can imagine. The ketogenic diet is most definitely not the best option for you if you realize that you would not be able to live with such tight carbohydrate limits for years to come.

Restrict Carbohydrates

Restrict carbs on a specific low-carb or keto diet on twenty digestible gram per day or fewer. There is no reason to limit fiber; it may also be useful for ketosis.

Take High Fat Foods

To feel fulfilled, eat sufficient fat. A low-carb ketogenic diet is typically a higher-fat plan, so the nutrition you no longer get from sugar is provided by fat. This is the main difference between such a ketogenic diet and hunger, which often ends in ketosis. You are likely to feel exhausted and try to give up your food if you act as if you are hungry. A ketogenic diet, though, can help you stop being too hungry, make it sustainable and perhaps make you feel fantastic. So, eat sufficient protein-rich foods and low-carb vegetables to be satisfied, with enough extra fat. If you're constantly hungry, make sure that in most meals you get enough quantities of protein and, if not, add extra fat to your meals.

Maintain Protein Intake

Maintain a modest intake of proteins. A ketogenic diet is not supposed to be a diet with very high protein content. Despite fears that individuals consume "much more" protein on a ketogenic diet, this does not appear to be the case for most individuals. Since it is really large, most persons cannot overeat protein. While amino acids may be transformed to glucose from protein foods, only a limited proportion are converted under laboratory conditions. This may be due to human reasons, such as the degree of glucose resistance. However, even people with type 2 diabetes generally perform better with the appropriate amounts of protein prescribed by Nutrition Doctor if their diets are not low-carb.

Stop Snacking

When not craving, stop snacking. Consuming more frequently than you need, either eating for pleasure or consuming since there is something around, lowers ketosis and delays weight loss. Using keto snacks can reduce the harm between meals while you are hungry, so consider changing your meals and make snacks unnecessary.

Sleep More and Stop Stressing

Get adequate sleep and relieve tension. On balance, most individuals benefit from a minimum of 8 hours of sleep each night. But aim to keep under-control tension. Sleep deficiency and stress hormones increase blood sugar levels, delaying ketosis and fat loss. You can also find it challenging to adhere to a keto diet and avoid temptations.

Chapter 2: Getting Started with Ketogenic Diet

Prepare your attitude when you are planning your meals with a ketogenic diet. A significant transition is challenging to make, so worry about what is going to keep things on track. The best part of making significant adjustments to the system you eat is often coping with the responses of other people. At best, they might doubt your choice; at the very worst, with a package laden with processed carbs, they may show up at your door. Burning accumulated body fat for energy has its advantages. In patients with epilepsy, the keto diet has been shown to minimize attacks, and animal tests indicate that it could have anti-ageing, antibacterial, and cancer-fighting effects as well. Before you get to start with your ketogenic diet, here are some benefits of the ketogenic diet and a list of food to eat and to avoid. At the end of the chapter, there is a shopping list to ease your work and save your time.

2.1 Who can benefit from the Ketogenic Diet?

In order to treat some problems, a ketogenic diet may be an exciting option which could speed up weight loss. But it is challenging to obey, and meat and other fatty, refined, and salty foods, which are famously unhealthy, maybe healthy. We do not know much about the long-term consequences either, perhaps because it is too hard to stick to it for an extended period, people cannot eat this way. It is also important to note that increased mortality is associated with "yo-yo diets" that contribute to dramatic fluctuations in losing weight. Try to accept transition that is manageable for the long term instead of joining in the next common diet that will last only a few weeks or even months. The best proof for a long, healthy, lively life appears to be a nutritious, unpasteurized diet, abundant in very colourful and vegetables, fish, entire grains, almonds, beans, olive oil, and plenty of water.

2.2 Foods to Eat

Usually, a ketogenic diet reduces carbohydrates to 20–40 gram per day. Although this can seem difficult, many healthy foods will comfortably fit into this type of diet. Here are some balanced things to consume on a ketogenic diet.

Seafood

Fish are foods which are very keto-friendly. Shrimp and other fish, though practically carb-free, are abundant in B vitamins, calcium, and magnesium. The carbohydrates in various shellfish forms, however, differ. For example, seafood and most crabs do not include carbohydrates than other shellfish varieties do. As this seafood can still be used in a ketogenic diet, once you are attempting to remain within a small range, it is crucial to compensate for these carbohydrates.

Low-Carb Vegetables

In Low-Carbs vegetables, vitamin C and other nutrients, are poor in calories and carbohydrates yet rich in several vitamins. Veggies and other plants produce fibre, like most carbohydrates, the body does not digest and consume. The word "net carbs" literally refers to carbohydrates that the body consumes. There are relatively few net carbohydrates found in many vegetables. Nevertheless, eating one portion of "starchy" vegetables such as potatoes, beets can put you for the day over your total carbohydrate limit.

Cheese

Hundreds of varieties of cheese are available. Luckily, most of them are very low in carbohydrates and high in fat, making them a perfect match for a diet that is ketogenic. 1 gram of carbohydrates, 6 grams of protein, and a decent amount of calcium contains one ounce of cheese. Cheese is abundant in saturated fat, but the incidence of cardiovascular diseases has not been shown to rise. In fact, some studies indicate that cheese can help prevent heart disease. Furthermore, daily cheese consumption can help reduce muscle loss and vitality that happens with age.

Meat and Poultry

Poultry and meat on a keto diet are called staple foods. Fresh meat products are high in Vitamin B and other essential minerals and do not contain carbohydrates. They are also a perfect source of proteins, which during a deficient carb diet was shown to help maintain muscle mass. One research in older women showed that eating a diet rich in fatty meat resulted in five percent higher levels of HDL lipid than on a lower fat, high carbohydrates diet. Choosing grass-fed beef is safest, if possible. This is because grass-eating animals grow meat with higher levels of omega-3 fatty acids, oleic acid and antioxidants than grain-fed meat products.

Avocado

Avocados are incredibly healthy; nine grams of carbohydrates are found in 3 ounces, or around half of a large avocado. Seven of these, though, are fibre, so only 2 grams is its total carbohydrate count. Avocados are rich in many minerals and vitamins that many people do not get enough of, like potassium, an essential mineral. In comparison, excessive content of potassium will help make it easier to switch to a keto diet. Additionally, avocados may help raise levels of cholesterol and triglycerides.

Other Foods to Eat

Fatty fish: herring, wild-caught salmon and mackerel.

Eggs: pastured, organic whole eggs.

Full- fat cheese: cheddar, brie, mozzarella, goat cheese and cream cheese.

Meat: pork, venison, organ meats, grass-fed beef, and bison.

Full-fat dairy: butter, yoghurt, and cream.

Condiments: salt, fresh herbs, pepper, lemon juice, vinegar and spices.

Nuts and seeds: pumpkin seeds, macadamia nuts, walnuts, almonds, peanuts and flaxseeds.

Non-starchy vegetables: tomatoes, greens, broccoli, mushrooms and peppers.

Poultry: chicken and turkey.

Nut butter: almond, natural peanut, and cashew butter.

Healthy fats: avocado oil, coconut oil, coconut butter, olive oil and sesame oil.

2.3 Foods to Avoid

The primary aim of a ketogenic diet is to induce dietary ketosis, a physiological condition where, instead of carbs and sugar, your body burns processed fat for power. Here are some foods that you have to avoid in the ketogenic diet.

Beverages

As beverages are also a significant source of invisible sugars and carbohydrates, pay particular attention to what you consume. The bulk of your fluid intake should come from drink, and you should consume 5 to 8 cups of water a day. When practising Atkins Keto, the below drinks can be avoided:

- Mocha
- Non-light beers
- Colas
- Hot Chocolate
- Sweetened iced tea
- Frappuccino
- Ginger Ale
- Fruit juices
- Lemonade
- Grape Soda
- Root Beer
- Energy Drinks
- Sports Drinks
- Tonic Water
- Vitamin Water

- Cocktails

Grains

It is easy to reduce your carbohydrate intake to get the rest of your daily calories, the secret to a healthy ketogenic diet. The concern with grains is that they are packed with carbs that can damage the success of your dieting. If necessary, it is better to avoid grains entirely, including these:

- Barley
- Rice
- Quinoa
- Sorghum
- Pumpernickel
- Buckwheat
- Sandwich wraps
- Oatmeal
- White
- Oats
- Corn
- Flour and corn tortillas
- Sourdough
- Wheat
- Rye

Vegetables

The general keto rule is to stop all veggies growing below the ground when it comes to veggies. As they produce the most carbohydrates, avoid veggies with higher nutritional content. It is best to eat about 15g of net vegetable carbohydrates per day, and here are the ketogenic diet vegetables to avoid:

- Parsnips
- Cassava (Yucca)
- Potatoes
- Corn
- Artichoke
- Sweet potatoes
- Yams
- Peas
- Baked potatoes

Proteins

It is essential for retaining muscle mass to provide sufficient protein consumption on a ketogenic diet. Two excellent sources of protein that are poor in carbohydrates are seafood and poultry. You usually tend to go for higher-fat cuts of meat such as ribeye sausages, chicken breasts, and oily fish such as salmon on a ketogenic diet. A piece of advice would be to avoid or restrict processed meats, particularly:

- Other processed meats
- Breaded meats
- Bacon with added sugar

Legumes

Usually, leguminous plants like peas and beans are rich in protein and other essential nutrients. But they are another form of keto diet food to stop because they are high in carbohydrates:

- Lima beans
- Navy beans
- Baked beans

- Cannellini beans
- Great Northern beans
- Chickpeas
- Green peas
- Kidney beans
- Lima beans
- Black-eyed peas
- Lentils
- Pinto beans
- Black beans

Fruits

Although seeing fruits appear on a "food products to prevent on keto" list may sound a little surprising, some fruits are full of sugar and carbohydrates. Looking for low sugars fruits such as blueberries, strawberries, raspberries, blackberries, and tomato is your best option. Olives and avocados are excellent sources of good fat as well. It is best to stop fruits like:

- Fruit smoothies
- All fruit juices
- Tangerines
- Peaches
- Mangos
- Nectarines
- Dried fruits
- Grapes
- Fruit Juices

- Oranges

- Apples

- Pears

- Pineapples

- Bananas

Dairy

Dairy, when consumed in moderation, is usually a low carbohydrate food category. It is important to note, though, that milk does contain carbohydrates, so aim to restrict your consumption to no more than 5 ounces a day. Here are some milk foods that you can stop on keto:

- Creamed cottage cheese

- Condensed milk

- Fat-free or low-fat yoghurt

- Most kinds of milk

Oil and Unhealthy Fats

It is an integrated component of Atkins and another ketogenic diet to eat a reasonable amount of fat. While these oils can be carbohydrate-free, 4 teaspoons daily are the optimal consumption for additional fats.

2.4 Shopping List for Ketogenic Diet

Here is the essential shopping list before you start your ketogenic diet.

Produce

- avocado

- lime

- mushrooms

- romaine or leaf lettuce
- cherry tomatoes
- garlic
- green cabbage
- red bell pepper
- spinach
- green onions
- white onion

Proteins

- breakfast sausage
- bacon
- ground beef
- boneless, skinless chicken breasts

Eggs and Dairy

- blue cheese
- salted butter
- whole-milk yoghurt
- cream cheese
- eggs

Staples

- monk fruit extract
- almond butter
- vanilla extract
- almond flour
- soy sauce

- cocoa powder
- chicken broth
- coconut cream

Spices and Oils

- sesame seeds
- avocado oil
- garlic powder
- coconut oil
- sesame oil
- salt
- ground ginger
- cinnamon
- pepper

So when you know what to buy for your daily keto-friendly meals, you can save your time and energy that you were going to waste to prepare a list for your weekly shopping.

Chapter 3: Delicious Asian Ketogenic Soups and Broth Recipes

3.1 Chinese Keto Soups and Broth Recipes

Chinese Keto Hot and Sour Soup

Cooking Time: 50 minutes

Serving Size: 8

Calories: 369

Ingredients:

- 70 oz. water
- 1 oz. dried shiitake mushrooms
- 1 onion (cut in half)
- 1 carrot
- 2 whole eggs (beaten)
- 1 piece of ginger
- 1 lb. chicken
- 6 oz. bamboo shoots
- 1 red bell pepper

Spices:

- salt to taste
- green onion
- 1 fresh chilli pepper
- 2 teaspoon paprika powder
- 4 teaspoon locust bean gum powder
- 5 tablespoon rice vinegar

- 1 teaspoon white pepper
- 1 piece of fresh ginger
- 1 garlic clove
- 4 tablespoon (gluten-free) soy sauce

Method:

1. With the onion and the thumb-sized slice of ginger chopped into pieces, boil the chicken for approximately 30-40 minutes, depending on which chicken pieces size you use.

2. Cut the bell pepper, carrot, bamboo shoots, and mushrooms into small pieces as the chicken is boiling, and set aside.

3. Chop the chilli pepper and the ginger and garlic cloves into rough bits.

4. Along with some coarse-grained salts and pestle, add the chilli, ginger, and garlic into a mixer until you get a smooth chilli paste.

5. In a griddle or wide pan with a little oil, fry the shiitake mushrooms for 4-5 minutes, until golden brown.

6. Remove the chicken and ginger's bits and onion from the pot after the chicken is cooked long enough.

7. Hold the chicken broth in the pot, then remove the bits of ginger and onion.

8. Strip the meat from the bones of the chicken and cut it into small bits.

9. Transfer to the pot the sliced vegetables as well.

10. Add chilli paste, rice vinegar, paprika powder, white pepper, and soy sauce and stir well.

11. Sprinkle salt and stir. For 10-15 minutes, continue to cook.

12. In a cup, beat the two eggs and stir the soup in circular movements before you make a whirl.

13. When proceeding to stir, dump the pounded eggs into the soup.

14. Before continuing to the next step, let it simmer for 1-2 minutes. Add a reasonable volume of thickening agents that would be keto-friendly.

15. Let them boil and stir until the consistency of the soup is slightly dense.

16. Serve the soup, garnished with a little sliced green onion, instantly.

Chinese Style Drop-Egg Soup

Cooking Time: 8 minutes

Serving Size: 2

Calories: 230

Ingredients:

- ¼ teaspoon Salt
- 2 Cans Chicken Broth
- 2 Eggs
- ¼ teaspoon Xanthan Gum
- 1 Stalk Green Onion
- ½ teaspoon Soy Sauce
- ¼ teaspoon White Pepper

Method:

1. Collect all the ingredients.

2. Heat the chicken broth over moderate heat in a large stove-top oven. Bring to a boil, add soy sauce, cinnamon, sea salt, and xanthan gum.

3. Meanwhile, in a bowl, beat the eggs.

4. Chop the green onions finely and set them aside.

5. Turn off the heat as chicken broth completes a boil and instantly stream eggs into the pot while gently swirling soup in a circle.

6. In bowls with ladle broth, top with green onions, and serve warm!

Keto Wonton Soup

Cooking Time: 30 minutes

Serving Size: 8

Calories: 125

Ingredients:

- ½ cup bean sprouts
- ¼ cup green onions (sliced)
- 8 cups no-sodium chicken stock
- 4 ounces spinach
- ½ cup (sliced) mushrooms
- 1 pound lean ground pork
- 2 cloves garlic (finely chopped)
- ½ teaspoon salt
- 2 tablespoon coconut amino
- 1 tablespoon sesame oil
- 1 tablespoon ginger (finely chopped)

- ¼ teaspoon pepper

Method:

1. In a large pan, put the bone broth or chicken broth to a boil.

2. Meanwhile, mix the minced pork with the coconut, seasonal fat, garlic, ginger, and salt.

3. Drop 1 tablespoon of meatballs from the pork paste into the broth when the broth is heating.

4. For 3-4 minutes, cook.

5. Include the mushrooms and spinach, which are finely cut. Enable another 2 minutes to boil.

6. Season with pepper and salt and garnish.

Chinese Pork Egg Roll Soup

Cooking Time: 30 minutes

Serving Size: 6

Calories: 255

Ingredients:

- 6 cups chicken broth
- 1 tablespoon soy sauce
- green onions (chopped)
- toasted sesame seeds
- Sriracha
- 1 ½ teaspoons grated ginger
- small head green cabbage (shredded)

- 1 pound ground pork

- ½ teaspoon salt

- ½ teaspoon pepper

- 1 teaspoon sesame oil

- 1 yellow onion (diced)

- 1 orange bell pepper

- 4 cloves garlic (minced)

Method:

1. Cook the minced pork on medium-high heat until just cooked, using a big container. Drain the fat if necessary.

2. Add onion, Sesame oil, garlic, bell pepper, and ginger to the pot. Sauté for five minutes or until partially translucent onions become visible.

3. Replace the broth, soy sauce, lettuce, salt, and black pepper. To combine, blend well.

4. Bring the soup to a low boil and steam until the cabbage is wilted or for 20 minutes.

5. Season more into additional pepper and salt if needed.

6. Top with diced green onions and baked sesame seeds in each bowl. Per person serving, add a squirt of Sriracha for a little seasoning.

Chinese Chicken Soup

Cooking Time: 40 minutes

Serving Size: 8

Calories: 325

Ingredients:

- 1.5 cups (diced) celery
- Salt to taste
- Cilantro and (chopped) scallions
- 1 lb. baby spareribs
- 1 packet Coconut Herbal Packet
- 3 lbs. whole chicken
- 1.5 cups (diced) carrots
- 6-8 cups water

Method:

1. Add the carrots, chicken, spareribs, celery, if used, and one traditional herbal packet in a 6-quart pressure cooker.
2. Fill the pot with that much water, 6–10 cups, only to cover the whole chicken.
3. Seal the handle and lid.
4. Set for 50 minutes at high pressure. Allow the soup to release its natural strain.
5. Cook on a low heat for 10 hours or up to 24 hours for a slow cooker.
6. Take the ingredients to a flame in a soup pot for the stovetop, lower the heat and cook for 1 ½ to 2 hours. To

adjust for cooling, you may need to add a little more water.

7. Season salt. If necessary, add garnish before serving.

Chinese Beef Noodles Soup

Cooking Time: 30 minutes

Serving Size: 4

Calories: 220

Ingredients:

For the broth:

- 1-inch piece of habanero
- 1 teaspoon granulated sugar substitute
- ½ teaspoon sesame oil
- 1 tablespoon lime juice
- salt and pepper to taste
- 1 piece of lime peel
- 2 tablespoon sugar-free fish sauce
- 1 teaspoon black bean paste
- 1 clove garlic (minced)
- 2-inch ginger (peeled and chopped)
- 6 cups beef broth

For the soup:

- 2 Tablespoon chilli peppers (sliced)
- Fresh lime to garnish
- ½ cup shiitake mushrooms (thinly sliced)
- 1 lb. lean beef (thinly sliced)

- ½ cup scallions, thinly sliced
- ½ cup fresh cilantro (chopped)
- 2 packs zero carb noodles
- ½ cups (shredded) cabbage

Method:

1. For the broth: In a moderate soup cup, heat the sesame oil.
2. Add the paste of beans, garlic, ginger, and peel of a lime and braise for a minute or until aromatic.
3. Add (if using) fish sauce, chicken stock, and habanero.
4. Simmer for at least thirty minutes, possibly longer, to produce the best taste.
5. Strain the bits out so that only the broth is left.
6. To the broth, add the sugar replacement and the lemon juice. Season to taste to your sweet and salty preferences.
7. To make the soup: Divide the slices of noodles, cabbage, meat, mushrooms, coriander, scallions, and chilli pepper between four large bowls of soup.
8. Bring the broth to a boil and transfer it over the soup ingredients. Let it rest for 5 minutes and serve.

Keto Wonton-Less Soup

Cooking Time: 30 minutes

Serving Size: 10

Calories: 260

Ingredients:

The Meatballs

- 2 green onions (chopped)
- 1 large pastured egg
- 1 ½ pounds ground pork
- 1 teaspoon fish sauce
- 1 teaspoon grated fresh ginger
- 3 tablespoons coconut amino
- ¼ teaspoon (crushed) red pepper flakes
- 2 cloves garlic (minced)
- 1 teaspoon gluten-free oyster sauce

For The Broth

- 1 bunch green onions
- 14-ounce bag of coleslaw mix
- 2 teaspoons (grated) fresh ginger
- ½ teaspoon (crushed) red pepper flakes
- 8 cups chicken stock
- 2 tablespoons coconut amino
- 2 tablespoons fish sauce
- 2 cups of water
- 2 tablespoons oyster sauce

- 5 large cremini mushrooms (thinly sliced)

Method:

1. Merge ground pork, red pepper, coconut amino, and 1 teaspoon Oyster sauce, sesame oil, ginger, fish sauce, green onions, garlic, and egg in a large mixing cup.

2. Mix until it is well blended. Shape the mixture into bite-sized meatballs.

3. Around 40 meatballs may yield it.

4. Heat and cook 2 tablespoons of sesame oil in a slow cooker or Dutch oven over medium-high heat.

5. Add meatballs to the pot.

6. Cook the meatballs until they have been crispy and golden brown all over.

7. Splash a little chicken stock in the pot if they tend to adhere. From the pot, remove the meatballs and set aside.

8. Add chicken stock, oyster sauce, amino coconut, water, fish sauce, ginger, and red pepper flakes to the pot.

9. Bring to a boil and then, to simmer, reduce heat to medium. For 10 minutes, boil.

10. Add to the soup the meatballs, mushrooms, and cabbage. Let it simmer an extra five minutes before serving.

Low Carb Chicken and Bok Choy Soup

Cooking Time: 10 minutes

Serving Size: 6

Calories: 174.2

Ingredients:

- 1 onion (chopped)
- 6 green onions (chopped)
- Salt and pepper
- 4 eggs (beaten)
- 3 ounces fresh spinach (shredded)
- 2 cups (diced) cooked chicken
- 8 ounces fresh mushrooms
- 8 cups Chicken Broth
- 2 pounds bok choy
- 2 tablespoons soy sauce
- 2 tablespoons oil
- 3 cloves garlic (minced)

Method:

1. Chop the bok choy, leaving the stalks apart from the stems.

2. Heat the oil in a soup pot and sauté the garlic, onion, stalks of bok choy, and mushrooms until nearly tender.

3. Add bok choy leaves, meat, broth, and soy sauce. Just get it to a boil.

4. Stir in the eggs gently. Stir in the green onions and spinach until the egg is set.

5. With pepper and salt, adjust the spice.

Asian Beef and Spinach Soup

Cooking Time: 25 minutes

Serving Size: 2

Calories: 651

Ingredients:

- 2 eggs (beaten)
- toasted sesame seeds
- 1 tablespoon sesame oil
- salt and pepper
- 8 oz. water
- 4 oz. fresh baby spinach
- 14.5 oz. canned beef broth
- 2 tablespoon soy sauce or tamari
- 1 teaspoon garlic (minced)
- 4 green onions (chopped)
- 1 lb. steak

Method:

1. In a wide pan, heat the sesame oil, then add the soy sauce, garlic, and scallions.
2. Meanwhile, add salt and pepper to the steak and prepare it on a griddle pan until medium heat.
3. Add beef broth and water to the first pan as the steak cooks. Get the baby spinach to a boil, and add it.
4. Erase the steak from heat, and let it rest.
5. In a small cup or mug, beat the eggs and then add them to the soup while continuously stirring.

6. Break the steak into tiny bits, take any extra fat off. Serve in bowls and add to the soup. Use toasted sesame seeds to flavoring.

Chicken Wonton Soup with Bok Choy

Cooking Time: 35 minutes

Serving Size: 4

Calories: 313

Ingredients:

Chicken Meatballs

- 3 scallions
- 1 teaspoon jalapeno (chopped)
- 1 pound ground chicken
- 1 tablespoon (grated) ginger
- 3 garlic cloves (minced)
- 1 ¼ teaspoon kosher salt
- 2 tablespoons lemongrass (chopped)
- 1 shallot- finely (chopped)

Broth

- Toasted sesame oil
- Fresh chilli slices
- 4 cups chicken broth
- Drizzle toasted sesame oil
- Fresh herbs
- 4 scallions (sliced)

- Pinch white pepper
- Salt to taste
- 3 cups bok choy

Method:

1. In a medium cup, put the ground chicken and the rest of the meatball ingredients and blend until well mixed, using wet hands.

2. Shape small cherry-walnut-shaped balls using wet hands, knowing that they will swell in the broth, and position them on a baking sheet lined with parchment.

3. In a large pan, heat the broth and add the scallions' white portions (or leeks).

4. Get it to a soft boil. Add a pinch of white pepper to taste, and add salt.

5. Add 10 raw meatballs to the broth and boil gently.

6. Boil the meatballs gently until cooked for about five minutes. Bear in mind that the smaller the meatballs, the quicker they cook.

7. They will float when done. Serve hot.

Moo Goo Gai Pan

Cooking Time: 25 minutes

Serving Size: 8

Calories: 215

Ingredients:

- 1 teaspoon ground ginger
- 2 green onions (sliced)

- 2 tablespoon Oil (divided)
- 8 oz. Shiitake mushrooms (washed and sliced)
- 1 tablespoon (Minced) garlic
- 1 teaspoon sesame oil
- 2 lb. Boneless chicken breast (sliced)
- 2 tablespoon Soy sauce
- ¼ teaspoon liquid stevia
- Salt and pepper
- 1 cup chicken broth (divided)
- 14.5 oz. canned baby corn (drained)
- 8 oz. canned bamboo shoots (drained)
- 2 cups broccoli florets
- 1 cup snow peas
- 8 oz. canned water chestnuts (drained)

Method:

1. Heat 1 tablespoons of oil over medium-high heat in a large pan or wok. Add salt and black pepper to the chicken, then add oil directly.

2. Brown the meat on either side for around 2-3 minutes. Remove and set aside from the pan.

3. Add the one tablespoon of oil and the chicken broth to the pan and stored over medium-high heat.

4. When the chicken broth continues to boil, add the broccoli and cook before the broccoli becomes light green. Add water chestnuts, snow peas, baby corn, mushrooms, and bamboo shoots.

5. Reduce the heat to low and simmer, occasionally stirring, for 5 more minutes.

6. Combine the stevia, garlic, soy sauce, sesame oil, and ginger in a small bowl before frying the vegetables.

7. Return the chicken to the pan, swirl and add the mixture of soy sauce and swirl again.

8. Cook until it is all hot, remove it from the heat, and stir in the green onions. Serve hot.

3.2 Japanese Keto Soups and Broth Recipes

Keto Japanese Onion Soup

Cooking Time: 6 hours

Serving Size: 3

Calories: 340

Ingredients:

- 2 green onions (sliced)
- Kosher salt, to taste
- 2 garlic cloves (smashed)
- 1 cup of mushrooms (sliced)
- 2 celery stalks
- 2 large carrots (peeled and quartered)
- 6 cups chicken stock
- 4 tablespoon butter
- 2 onions (peeled and quartered)

Method:

1. Add all ingredients to your slow cooker except green onions and ¾ pack sliced mushrooms.
2. Cook for 5 to 6 hours at low temperatures.
3. Pour slow cooker contents into a pot or large bowl via a strainer.
4. In the slow cooker, add liquid back in.
5. Add the chopped spring onions and the remainder of the mushrooms and slices.
6. Ladle it into a bowl and eat.

Keto Chicken Ramen Soup

Cooking Time: 2 hours 10 minutes

Serving Size: 4

Calories: 484

Ingredients:

- 1 small organic chicken
- 12 cups water
- 6 green onions (chopped)
- 4 tablespoon gluten-free soy sauce
- 2 tablespoon salt
- 2 packs of shirataki noodles
- 2 organic chicken broth cubes
- 4 large eggs

Method:

1. Bring the water to a boil in a big pot and add the chicken to it.

2. Transfer the chicken stock cubes and salt and lower the heat to medium-low.

3. Cover and cook for fifteen minutes and 1 hour.

4. Keep the broth uncovered and let it cook for another 45 minutes on low heat.

5. Remove the chicken from the water. Move through a strainer until the broth is ready to get clear of any particulates.

6. Rip the carcass of all its meat after the chicken has cooled down and put it in a pan.

7. Bring 4 cups of water to a boil in a medium pot and carefully put the 4 eggs in it. For perfectly runny egg yolks, cook for exactly 6 minutes.

8. Put half a pack of shirataki noodles, one tablespoon of soy sauce, as much chicken as you want, one half-cut soft boiled egg, and a handful of chopped green onions in each dish. Serve hot.

Japanese Clear Onion Soup

Cooking Time: 30 minutes

Serving Size: 6

Calories: 24

Ingredients:

- to taste soy sauce
- to taste Sriracha
- 1 cup button mushrooms (sliced)
- ½ cup scallions (sliced)
- 1 carrot (peeled and diced)
- 1 tablespoon garlic (minced)
- 1 teaspoon sesame oil
- to taste salt and pepper
- 6 cups vegetable broth
- 2 onions (chopped)
- 1 celery stalks (diced)
- ½ teaspoon ginger (minced)

Method:

1. In a pot, sauté the onions in a bit of oil until lightly caramelized. About ten minutes.

2. Put the carrot, garlic, celery, ginger, sesame oil, and broth in the mixture. Season with pepper and salt to taste.

3. Bring it to a boil and simmer for thirty minutes.

4. From the broth, strain the vegetables.

5. Attach a couple of bowls of scallions and finely sliced mushrooms. On top, ladle the broth.

6. Add a dash of soy sauce and sriracha sauce to taste.

Keto Pumpkin Soup

Cooking Time: 25 minutes

Serving Size: 6

Calories: 243.5

Ingredients:

- 1 teaspoon salt
- 1 cup heavy cream
- 2 tablespoons heavy cream
- 3 tablespoons (crushed) walnuts
- 2 ½ cups chicken stock
- 1 can pumpkin puree
- 2 tablespoons brown sugar
- 1 ½ teaspoons pumpkin pie spice
- 1 tablespoon olive oil
- 1 small onion (diced)

- 2 cloves garlic (minced)

Method:

1. Heat oil in a saucepan over medium heat. Add the onion and sauté for two or three minutes. Lower the heat to medium-low, then add the garlic.

2. Sauté for two to three more minutes, until the onion begins to soften. Stir in the sugar, pumpkin pie spice, and seasoning.

3. Pour in chicken stock and stir to blend. Whisk in the pumpkin puree, cover, and cook for ten minutes over medium-low heat.

4. Blend soup cautiously until smooth using an electric mixer.

5. Stir in one cup of heavy cream and modify seasoning, if necessary.

6. Garnish with heavy cream and chopped walnuts.

Vegan Thai Soup

Cooking Time: 25 minutes

Serving Size: 4

Calories: 339

Ingredients:

- The juice of half a lime
- A handful of fresh cilantro (chopped)
- ½ julienned red onion
- 10 oz. firm tofu (cubed)
- 1 tablespoon tamari or soy sauce

- 2 cups vegetable broth
- 1 14-ounce can coconut milk
- ½ julienned red bell pepper
- ½ inch piece of ginger root
- ½ Thai chilli (chopped)
- 3 sliced mushrooms
- 2 cloves of garlic (chopped)
- 1 tablespoon coconut

Method:

1. Place all the vegetables in a big pot (onion, garlic, ginger, red pepper, mushrooms, and Thai chilli pepper), stock, coconut milk, and sugar.

2. Bring it to a boil and then simmer for around five minutes over medium heat.

3. Insert the tofu and cook for an extra five minutes.

4. Connect the tamari, lime juice, and fresh cilantro and remove it from the sun. Mix and serve.

5. For up to five days, store the soup in a sealed jar in the refrigerator.

Life-Changing Chicken Udon

Cooking Time: 10 minutes

Serving Size: 1

Calories: 608

Ingredients:

- 1 dry udon noodles
- ½ green onion, (chopped)
- 2 cups dashi broth
- 1 tablespoon Sake
- ½ tablespoons. sugar
- 1 boneless
- ½ of a small leek
- 1 tablespoon soy sauce
- 1 tablespoon mirin

Method:

1. Combine the dashi broth, mirin, soy sauce, and sugar in a saucepan. Bring it to a boil and let it cook for two to three minutes.

2. Then, add sake, chicken thigh, and leek.

3. Stir to heat equally, bring the soup back to a simmer, then cook for approximately 3 minutes or until the chicken is fully cooked, and the leek is tender and nice.

4. By following the instructions of the packet you are using, cook the udon noodles. If you are using fresh frozen udon, when the chicken is almost finished, start cooking it.

5. If you are using a dry one that requires a few moments, then when you start to cook the chicken soup part, begin cooking the noodles.

6. Place the fried udon and spill the chicken soup into a serving dish. Sprinkle and serve directly with sliced green onion.

Miyabi Japanese Onion Soup

Cooking Time: 35 minutes

Serving Size: 10

Calories: 310

Ingredients:

- 1 mushroom (thinly sliced)
- 1 tablespoon onions
- 3 cups beef broth
- 2 garlic cloves (crushed)
- 1 green onion (thinly sliced)
- 1 large carrot
- 1 medium onion (chopped)
- 7 cups chicken broth

Method:

1. Take a bowl and mix beef and chicken stock.

2. Add the carrot, garlic, and onion.

3. Bring to a boil, cover, and simmer for thirty minutes.

4. Throw away the carrot, onion, and garlic, then filter the broth through the paper towel.

5. In serving bowls, put a small number of green onions, mushrooms, and french fried onions and ladle over them with the broth. Serve hot.

Chicken and White Bean Soup

Cooking Time: 40 minutes

Serving Size: 4

Calories: 345

Ingredients:

- 1 tablespoon white wine vinegar
- ¼ teaspoon salt
- 2 cups chicken broth
- ½ cup (uncooked) orzo
- 1 garlic clove (minced)
- 1 cup (chopped) plum tomato
- 2 tablespoons (chopped) fresh oregano
- 2 smoked bacon slices (chopped)
- 12 ounces chicken thighs
- ½ cup (chopped) onion
- ¼ teaspoon black pepper
- 2 cups of water
- 1 can organic white beans
- 2 tablespoons (chopped) flat-leaf parsley

Method:

1. Cook the bacon in a large saucepan for 10 minutes or until crispy, over medium heat.

2. Remove the bacon from the pan and reserve the drippings in the pan; set aside the bacon.

3. Add the chicken to the pan's drippings; sauté for 6 minutes.

4. Take the chicken from the casserole. Transfer the garlic and onion to the pan; cook for 4 minutes or until tender.

5. Add the tomato, oregano, and pepper; roast, stirring continuously, for two minutes.

6. Put the bacon and chicken back in the pan. Stir in two cups of broth and water and scrub the pan to loosen the browned bits. Just get it to a boil.

7. Insert the orzo and cook until browned, or for 10 minutes.

8. Add beans; cook until hot, or two minutes.

9. Stir in the parsley, vinegar, and salt. Remove from the heat.

Jalapeño Popper Soup

Cooking Time: 30 minutes

Serving Size: 6

Calories: 330

Ingredients:

- Pinch cumin
- 4 oz. Reduced-fat cream cheese

- 1 tablespoon butter
- ¼ teaspoon Garlic powder
- 3 tablespoon Flour
- 1 cup Corn
- ¼ teaspoon Onion powder
- ½ green bell pepper (diced)
- ¾ cup Whole milk
- ½ teaspoon Salt
- ½ onion (chopped)
- ¼ teaspoon Paprika
- ½ red bell pepper (diced)
- 3-4 jalapeño peppers (minced)
- 3 cloves garlic (minced)
- 1 head cauliflower (chopped)
- 3½ cup Chicken broth
- ¼ teaspoon Ground pepper
- ¼ teaspoon Chili powder

Garnishes (optional):

- Slices of jalapeño
- Cheddar cheese
- Bacon crumbles

Method:

1. Melt the butter over medium-low heat in a big stockpot or griddle.

2. Insert the bell peppers and onion and cook for around 3-4 minutes, until tender.

3. Connect the jalapeño peppers and the chopped garlic and simmer for another 1 minute.

4. Stir in the cauliflower and maize, cook for around 3-4 minutes, then sprinkle on top with the flour and cook until nicely browned.

5. Mix in the chicken broth and milk and cook until the mixture starts to boil. Switch the heat to low.

6. Include the seasonings and continue simmering until the cauliflower is crispy or for fifteen minutes.

7. Transfer the cream cheese and whisk until mixed vigorously.

8. Remove from the fire and garnish with the toppings you want. Immediately serve.

3.3 Thai Keto Soups and Broth Recipes

Thai Coconut Soup Recipe

Cooking Time: 35 minutes

Serving Size: 6

Calories: 227

Ingredients:

- 2 sprigs Thai basil fresh
- Cilantro to garnish
- 4 chicken breasts large
- 1 tablespoon coconut amino
- 1 oz. lime juice
- 1 teaspoon ground ginger
- 14 oz. coconut milk
- 14 oz. chicken broth
- 28 oz. water
- ¼ cup red boat fish sauce
- 2 tablespoon Thai garlic chilli paste

Method:

1. Finely chop the chicken breast into ¼ inch wide pieces, and cut again to produce bite-sized parts of the chicken.

2. Merge coconut milk, fish sauce, broth, water, chilli sauce, lime juice, amino coconut, ginger, and basil in a large stock container.

3. Carry it over high heat to a boil.

4. Stir in the pieces of chicken, reduce heat to medium-low and cover; simmer for thirty minutes.

5. Strip the basil leaves and garnish with coriander on the soup.

Keto Curry Soup

Cooking Time: 30 minutes

Serving Size: 4

Calories: 462

Ingredients:

- 1 tablespoon lime juice
- ½ tablespoon fish sauce
- 4 cups vegetable broth
- 1 can full-fat coconut milk
- 2 cups wild mushrooms (chopped)
- 1 tablespoon yellow curry paste
- 4 tablespoons ghee
- 1 small white onion (chopped)
- 1-inch piece of fresh ginger (minced)
- 1 serrano pepper (thinly sliced)
- 1 large carrot cut into rounds
- 3 cloves garlic (minced)

Method:

1. Heat ghee over medium-high heat in a big 5-quart Dutch oven.

2. Add the garlic, carrot, onion, ginger, and serrano once it is warmed.

3. Sauté for five minutes until the softening starts.

4. Put in the mushrooms and paste of curry, stir to blend and add in the rest of the ingredients.

5. Reduce the heat to a boil, cover and cook until the carrots are tender for another ten minutes.

6. Divide between 4 bowls for serving and top with the desired toppings.

Keto Thai Coconut Chicken Soup

Cooking Time: 50 minutes

Serving Size: 3

Calories: 320

Ingredients:

- 1 stalk lemongrass
- Cilantro to garnish
- 1 teaspoon ground ginger
- 2 Thai basil leaves
- 1 tablespoon soy sauce
- Juice from half of a small lime
- 1 lb. boneless skinless chicken thighs
- ¼ cup Red Boat fish sauce
- 1.5 tablespoon Sriracha
- 14 oz. can of coconut milk
- 2 cups chicken broth

- 3.5 cups water

Method:

1. Combine the coconut milk, chicken broth, and water over moderate heat in a large stockpot.

2. Add the Sriracha, lime juice, fish sauce, soy sauce (or coconut amino), garlic, and Thai basil.

3. Lemongrass preparation: slice the ends off, draw the rough outer coating off, and then cut the 1-inch strip at a diagonal angle. Add to the pot of stock.

4. Clean the thighs of the chicken and cut them into bite-sized bits.

5. Increase the heat to boil the stockpot mixture.

6. Then stir in the pieces of chicken, reduce the heat to medium-low, and cover the oven. For thirty minutes, boil.

7. Remove the lemongrass and basil from the soup.

Thai Chicken Zoodle Soup

Cooking Time: 30 minutes

Serving Size: 8

Calories: 277

Ingredients:

- 2 medium zucchini (spiralizer)
- 1 lime cut into 8 wedges
- 2 tablespoon fish sauce
- ¼ cup chopped cilantro
- 1 tablespoon coconut oil

- 1 medium red pepper (thinly sliced)
- 1 pound chicken breasts
- ¼ medium onion (chopped)
- 6 cups of chicken bone broth
- 13.5 ounces of canned coconut milk
- 1 jalapeño (chopped)
- 1 ½ tablespoon green curry paste
- 2 cloves garlic (minced)

Method:

1. Warm the coconut oil in a pan over medium heat until it is melted.

2. Add the onions, and heat for about five minutes until translucent.

3. Stir in the jalapeño, curry mixture and garlic, and sauté for around two minutes, until fragrant.

4. Add coconut milk and broth and mix until thoroughly mixed.

5. Lower the flame to moderate and add the red pepper, meat and fish sauce. Bring to a boil.

6. Leave to boil for another five minutes until the chicken is cooked through. Stir the coriander in.

7. Divide the zoodles among eight bowls of soup and ladle over the soup; the soup heat will make the zoodles tender.

8. With a squeeze of lime, serve each one.

Thai Coconut Curry Chicken Soup

Cooking Time: 30 minutes

Serving Size: 6

Calories: 223

Ingredients:

- 1 clove garlic (minced)
- 1 tablespoon butter
- Keto-friendly mild-flavored oil
- 12 ounces chicken breast (shredded)
- juice of 1 lime
- 1 tablespoon fresh cilantro
- 2 tablespoons red curry paste
- 1 tablespoon scallions (sliced)
- 2 teaspoons ginger (grated)
- 6 cups chicken stock
- 1 tablespoon fish sauce
- 2-inch piece lemongrass
- 5 ounces shiitake mushrooms (sliced)
- 13.5-ounce coconut milk
- 1 small zucchini (sliced)
- ½ cup red pepper (sliced)

Method:

1. The chicken is prepared by shredding the cooked chicken breast.
2. Take the lemongrass portion and strike it with the back of your knife a couple of times.

3. Heat a big pot to moderate, add oil and butter and sauté for several minutes with the mushrooms and red pepper.

4. Add the garlic and ginger and sauté for about 20 seconds, then stir in the curry paste and simmer for ten seconds until toasted.

5. Deglaze the pot with the chicken stock.

6. Insert the chicken, lime juice, fish sauce, lemongrass and scallions to the coconut milk.

7. Boil, uncovered, for fifteen minutes. Add the zucchini and let it cook for another five minutes or until tender.

8. Garnish with clean cilantro, discard the lemongrass and serve with a squeeze of lime

9. Store the leftovers in the refrigerator or freezer for several days.

Thai Chicken and Vegetable Soup

Cooking Time: 50 minutes

Serving Size: 4

Calories: 194

Ingredients:

- 1 oz. of (chopped) cilantro
- 1 lime (quartered)
- 2 tablespoons of olive oil
- 1 medium zucchini
- 4 oz. of bean shoots
- 8 oz. of (shredded) cooked chicken

- 1 (sliced) red pepper
- 4 cups of chicken broth
- 2 oz. of snow peas
- ½ a cup of coconut milk
- ½ (diced) red onion
- 3 (chopped) green onions
- 2 tablespoons of red Thai curry paste

Method:

1. In a big saucepan, heat the oil.
2. In a hot pan, add the red onion and fry until it starts to brown.
3. Add the curry paste and the spring onions, and fry.
4. Insert the bell peppers after several minutes and fry them for two more minutes.
5. Pour the chicken broth into the mixture and simmer for fifteen minutes.
6. Now add the bean shoots, snow peas, and cooked shredded chicken and boil five minutes slowly.
7. Insert the zoodles and let them cook for another two minutes.
8. Stir in the milk of coconut and release it from the heat.
9. Dish up and serve with a dash of mint, cilantro, and a lime slices.

Thai Hot and Sour Shrimp Soup

Cooking Time: 55 minutes

Serving Size: 2

Calories: 246

Ingredients:

- ¼ bunch fresh Thai basil (chopped)
- Salt and pepper, to taste
- 2 tablespoon fish sauce
- ¼ bunch fresh cilantro (chopped)
- 1 small green zucchini
- 5 cups chicken broth
- ½ lb. oyster or button mushrooms
- 2 tablespoon fresh lime juice
- 3 each fresh kaffir lime leaves
- 1 one inch ginger root
- 1 each lemongrass stalk
- 1 red and green Thai chillies (rough chop)
- 1 lb. shrimp (peeled)
- 2 tablespoon coconut oil (divided)
- 1 medium onion (diced)
- 4 each garlic cloves

Method:

1. Chop the shrimp and devein it, leaving aside the shrimp shells.

2. Warm coconut oil over a moderate flame in a big pan. Add the shells of the shrimp and mix rapidly to cook them.

3. Cook until the color is red and any ammonia scent is lost.

4. Add the garlic, onion, ginger, lemongrass, lime leaves, chillies, and a little bit of salt and pepper, or a slight amount of fresh lime zest.

5. Cook until the onions are mildly transparent, or around three minutes. Transfer the chicken broth to the casserole and boil.

6. Strain it until the shrimp supply has simmered for around thirty minutes. Over the high fire, heat a large sauté pan.

7. When hot, sprinkle a little bit of salt and pepper to the coconut oil, zucchini and mushrooms.

8. Sauté until thoroughly cooked, but still marginally firm. Add the shrimp stock to it. To the shrimp broth, insert the raw shrimp.

9. For around 2 minutes, enable the veggies and shrimp to boiling. Insert the lime juice, sauce and a sprinkle of salt and pepper.

10. Flavor the broth and change the seasoning. When the shrimp is ready, add the fresh cilantro and basil.

11. Heat for an extra 1 minute. Serve hot.

Thai Shrimp and Veggie Soup

Cooking Time: 20 minutes

Serving Size: 10

Calories: 211

Ingredients:

- ¼ cup Lime Juice
- 1 tablespoon Soy Sauce
- 1 teaspoon Fish Sauce
- Red pepper flakes
- ½ cup (frozen) bell pepper pieces
- 4 Cups Chicken Broth
- 14 oz. Coconut milk (canned)
- 1 tablespoon butter
- 8 oz. Sliced Mushrooms White
- 3 inch Ginger
- ½ cup Green Onion
- 1 teaspoon garlic
- ½ Cup Sliced Celery
- 4 cups Bok Choy (Chopped)
- 1 teaspoon black pepper
- 1 pound Shrimp

Method:

1. Sauté the ginger and celery for three minutes in a wide casserole dish as you cut the bok choy.

2. When starting to sauté, add peppers, mushrooms and onions.

3. Add bok choy, then begin to sauté.

4. Add the chicken broth, garlic, fish sauce, soya sauce, pepper, and coconut milk until the mushrooms begin to darken. Bring it to a boil.

5. Add the shrimp and boil for about 3 minutes underneath the liquid or until the pink and vegetables are cooked but still a little crisp.

6. Turn the heat off and add some lime juice.

7. Serve with red pepper flakes and cilantro.

Thai Peanut Curry Squash Soup

Cooking Time: 35 minutes

Serving Size: 8

Calories: 128

Ingredients:

- ¼ cup Cilantro (Chopped)
- Sriracha optional for garnish
- 5 cups Butternut Squash (seeded and cubed)
- 1 teaspoon Fish Sauce
- ¼ cup (Chopped) Peanuts
- 2 tablespoon Natural Peanut Butter
- ¼ Yellow Onion (chopped)
- 1 teaspoon Ground Ginger
- 2 tablespoon Red Curry Paste
- 4 cups Chicken Broth
- 13.5 oz. Can Coconut Milk

- ½ teaspoon Garlic Powder

Method:

1. Add in the instant pot all of the ingredients excluding peanuts and cilantro.

2. Set the steam release valve to be shut by placing the lid on the instant pot.

3. Use the manual setting and cook under high pressure for 10 minutes. Enable to steam, then open the lid, to release normally.

4. To puree the squash and all the components together, use an electric mixer.

5. When desired, serve topped with peanuts, Sriracha and cilantro.

Low Carb Keto Pho

Cooking Time: 34 minutes

Serving Size: 4

Calories: 218

Ingredients:

Pho Broth

- 1 tablespoon Bestir Monk Fruit Allulose Blend
- Sea salt
- 4 whole Star anise
- 8 cups beef bone broth
- 1 tablespoon Fish sauce
- 2 whole Cardamom pods

- 1 tablespoon Coriander seeds

- 1 teaspoon ground ginger

- 2 whole Cinnamon sticks

- 2 whole Cloves

Pho Soup

- 2 large Zucchini

- 12 oz. Flank steak

Optional Pho Toppings

- Scallions

- Sriracha

- Thai basil

- Red chilli pepper slices

- Cilantro

- Lime Wedges

Method:

1. To make it easy to slice finely, put the steak in the freezer for thirty minutes.

2. In the meantime, heat a casserole dish over medium-high heat, with no oil.

3. Add star anise, cubes of cardamom, sticks of cinnamon, cloves, seeds of coriander and ground ginger. Give 3 minutes of toast, until fragrant.

4. Add the fish sauce and bone broth. Stir continuously. Boil the pho broth and simmer for thirty minutes.

5. In the meantime, use a spiralizer to make zoodles out of the zucchini. Divide the zucchini noodles among four cups.

6. Take it out and cut very thinly against the grain once the steak in the freezer is firm. Position the steak in each bowl on top of the zoodles.

7. Stir in the sugar substitute to dissolve and change the salt to taste when the broth is finished simmering.

8. Through another pot or pan, strain the broth. Dispose of the whole spices caught in the strainer.

9. While broth is still boiling, immediately pour it over the prepared pots, making sure that you submerge the steak so that it roasts through. Serve with toppings of choice.

Chapter 4: Asian Comfort Food and Spicy Tasty Dishes

This chapter will cover the Asian comfort foods and spicy foods that will keep you warm in winter with delicious taste and readily available ingredients.

4.1 High Protein Winter Comfort Food Recipes

Creamy Sundried Tomato and Parmesan Chicken Zoodles

Cooking Time: 30 minutes

Serving Size: 6

Calories: 394

Ingredients:

- Red chilli flakes
- 2 large Zucchini
- Salt to taste
- (Dried) basil seasoning
- 1 tablespoon butter
- 300 ml thickened cream
- 1 cup (shaved) Parmesan cheese
- 100 g sun-dried tomatoes in oil (chopped)
- 4 cloves garlic (peeled and crushed)
- 700g skinless chicken thigh fillets
- 120 g fresh semi-dried tomato

Method:

1. Melt the butter over medium-low heat in a pan. Insert strips of chicken and spray with seasoning.

2. Pan Fry until both sides of the chicken are golden brown and heated through.

3. Add a small tablespoon of oil from the bottle to both semi-dried and sun-dried tomatoes and add the garlic; sauté until

4. Transfer the cream and cheese to the lower heat; boil when stirring until the cheese has melted.

5. To your preference, brush over the flour, basil and red chilli flakes.

6. Stir via the zoodles and proceed to boil until the zoodles (about 8 minutes) has softened to your taste and serve.

Cauliflower Mac and Cheese

Cooking Time: 20 minutes

Serving Size: 4

Calories: 350

Ingredients:

- 2 tablespoons olive oil
- 16-ounce cauliflower florets
- (freshly ground) black pepper
- ¼ cup parmesan cheese (finely grated)

Cheese Sauce:

- ½ teaspoon garlic powder
- ¼ teaspoon ground cayenne
- ½ cup heavy whipping cream

- 2 teaspoons Dijon mustard
- ½ teaspoon table salt
- 1 cup (shredded) cheddar cheese
- 2 ounces cream cheese (chopped)

Method:

1. Cauliflower Roast: Preheat the oven to 400F. If the florets of cauliflower are exceeding 2 inches, cut them into tiny chunks.

2. On the foil-lined baking plate, toss the florets with coconut oil until well-coated, then scatter the florets in a single layer.

3. Bake for 20 minutes at 400 F till tender. Proceed to the next stage of cooking the sauce when baking.

4. Make Sauce: In a medium bowl, mix all the sauce components over medium-high heat until molten and smooth, around 5 minutes, reducing heat as required, so that the sauce is not hot enough to boil.

5. Keep warm over low heat until mixed while waiting for the cauliflower to roast.

6. Serve: In a mixing cup, toss the roasted cauliflower with the sauce until well covered.

Shakshuka (Eggs in Tomato Sauce)

Cooking Time: 30 minutes

Serving Size: 3

Calories: 520

Ingredients:

- 2 tablespoons olive oil
- Freshly ground black pepper
- Crusty bread (for serving)
- ½ cup yellow onion (chopped)
- ¼ cup fresh parsley (chopped)
- 3 large eggs
- 1 cup sweet red pepper (diced)
- 3 cups (chopped) tomatoes
- 1 teaspoon salt
- 2 tablespoons garlic (minced)

Method:

1. Over medium-high heat, heat the heating oil in a deep fryer or stainless steel skillet.

2. Insert the onions and diced peppers and cook for about ten minutes, stirring regularly, until the onion becomes translucent and the red pepper lightens.

3. To combine all the ingredients, add salt, seasoning and tomato and stir well.

4. Continue cooking until the mixture thickens, around twenty minutes.

5. Stir in the parsley that has been sliced. Crack the eggs straight into the sauce one at a time, reduce the heat to medium and cover the pan.

6. Remove from the heating when the eggs have a soft coat of white over the yolks.

7. Add a few shreds of black pepper and insert some chopped fresh parsley to the combination. Serve hot with bread and eat it.

Low Carb Keto Philly Cheesesteak Stuffed Peppers with Cauliflower

Cooking Time: 50 minutes

Serving Size: 6

Calories: 379

Ingredients:

For The Onions:

- Salt

- 2 large onions (sliced) about ½ thick

- 1 tablespoon Olive oil

For The Peppers:

- Salt

- 12 oz. provolone cheese (shredded)

- 6 Small green bell peppers

- 1 tablespoon olive oil

- 2 cups cauliflower

- 1 lb. beef top sirloin steak

Method:

1. Heat 1 tablespoon of olive oil in a wide pan over medium heat until smooth.

2. Add sliced onions to it. And a pinch of salt, swirling until it is coated with grease.

3. Cook, stirring periodically, till the onions are nicely browned and caramelized, for 30-45 minutes.

4. Place the ready peppers in a big pot when the onions are cooking and cover them with water.

5. Bring to a boil and simmer for 3 minutes, until just softened.

6. Drain and put, softly patting some of the water off, on a sheet of paper towel. In a 9x13 inch pan, place the peppers, and switch the 350 degrees.

7. Heat the remaining 1 tablespoon of oil over medium heat in a wide pan.

8. Cook the grilled steak until golden brown. Shift to a dish.

9. Put the cauliflower in a big hand blender when the beef is cooking.

10. Place it right in the pan that the beef was in and process on medium-high heat, stirring regularly until lightly browned.

11. When the beef and caramelized onions are cooked, add them to the pan and sprinkle them with sea salt. Stir before it is blended properly.

12. With the combination, stuff the peppers and cover each pepper with a cheese slice.

13. Bake for about 15 minutes, until the cheese is molten and the peppers are tender.

14. Switch the oven to a strong broiler and cook till the cheese is nicely browned for another 4 minutes. Serve hot.

4.2 Low Carbs Spicy Dishes to keep you Warm

Keto Low Carb Gluten-Free Chicken and Dumplings Recipe

Cooking Time: 30 minutes

Serving Size: 8

Calories: 273

Ingredients:

- 2 medium (Dried) bay leaves
- ½ recipe fathead bagel dough
- 1 tablespoon olive oil
- 1 ½ lb. chicken breast
- 8 cups chicken broth
- 1 stalk celery
- 2 tablespoon Italian seasoning
- ½ large onion
- 1 large carrot

Method:

1. Place to sauté the Instant Pot on the flame. Add onion, celery, carrots and olive oil. Sauté before tender, for about ten minutes.

2. Add the spice. Sauté till scented.

3. Add the chicken, chicken stock and basil leaves. Cover the lid and lock it.

4. Set five minutes to manual high pressure. Use fast release to release the pressure when the soup is finished cooking.

5. Meanwhile, produce fathead dough according to the same recipes and proportions as the recipe for fathead bagels, except that the recipe is divided in half.

6. If the dough is moist, refrigerate it until solid, for around twenty minutes.

7. Place between two sheets of oiled parchment paper with the fathead dough.

8. Remove the lid until the soup is ready and the pressure is removed.

9. Remove the chicken and slice the bits (or shreds) into bite sizes. Return to the pot.

10. Then, switch the instant pot to sauté function. Add dumplings and stir for about three minutes, until fully cooked.

Low-Carb Lasagna Chicken Recipe

Cooking Time: 35 minutes

Serving Size: 4

Calories: 420

Ingredients:

- ½ cup (shredded) mozzarella cheese
- 2 tablespoon fresh basil
- ¼ teaspoon pepper
- 4 boneless chicken breasts
- 2 tablespoon (grated) Parmesan cheese
- ½ cup marinara sauce
- ¼ cup ricotta cheese

- 1 large egg
- 2 tablespoon olive oil
- ½ teaspoon salt

Method:

1. Preheat the oven to 375 degrees.

2. Place the chicken breasts minimum 1 inch apart on a sheet dish. Brush the chicken with oil on both ends. With pepper and salt, season all ends.

3. Put the ricotta and egg together in such a small tub, then whisk in the Parmesan.

4. Spread uniformly over the breasts of chicken.

5. Put two tablespoons of marinara sauce to each slice of chicken, then brush with two tablespoons of mozzarella.

6. Bake for 23 to 28 minutes, until thoroughly cooked.

Cauliflower Fried Rice Recipe

Cooking Time: 32 minutes

Serving Size: 4

Calories: 452

Ingredients:

- 1 teaspoon Sriracha
- Lime wedges (for serving)
- 1 head cauliflower
- ¼ cup (chopped) Thai basil
- 1-3 tablespoon soy sauce

- 1 cup shredded carrots (roughly chopped)
- 1 cup frozen peas
- 5 slices thick-cut bacon (chopped)
- 1 pound organic chicken breast
- 3 large eggs (beaten)
- 3 cloves (minced) garlic
- 1 bunch green onions (chopped)
- 1 tablespoon (freshly grated) ginger
- Coconut oil, for frying

Method:

1. Slice the bacon, meat, and veggies. In the mixing bowl, split the cauliflower into florets and position them. Pulse until it resembles grain, loosely.

2. Over medium fire, heat a large skillet. Place the covered dish as a storage dish on the side of the wok.

3. To the pan, add the bacon and cook until nicely browned. With a slotted spoon, cut and put in the bowl.

4. Add the skillet with the eggs and fry quickly. To split it into tiny pieces, use your spoon, then switch to the holding dish.

5. Add a little bit of oil to the wok, if necessary.

6. Add the chicken, white onion bits, garlic, and ginger and turn the fire up to high.

7. Fry till the meat is barely finished, then add the carrots and fry for another minute. Switch to the storage dish using a slotted spoon.

8. Now transfer the "rice" cauliflower to the skillet. Stir fry until smooth, but still solid, for 5 minutes.

9. Return all the cooked items to the skillet, along with the peas, sauce and chilli paste, to taste.

10. Toss and roast, then toss in the green onion tops until the peas are heated through. With lime slices, serve hot.

Easy Szechuan Beef Recipe

Cooking Time: 20 minutes

Serving Size: 6

Calories: 329

Ingredients:

For the Stir Fry Sauce:

- 6 cloves garlic (minced)
- 1 tablespoon Szechuan peppercorns
- 2 tablespoons brown sugar
- 2 tablespoons (fresh grated) ginger
- 2 tablespoons hoisin sauce
- 2 tablespoons mirin rice wine
- ¼ cup (low sodium) soy sauce
- 3 tablespoons water

For the Beef:

- 1 tablespoon sesame oil
- 1 bunch scallions
- 1 tablespoon sesame seeds
- 1 ½ pound flat iron stock
- 2 tablespoon peanut oil

- 12 whole (dried) Szechuan Chile peppers
- 1 ½ tablespoon cornstarch

Method:

1. Transfer all of the items for the stir-fry sauces to a liquid mixing bowl. Cut and put the scallions aside.

2. Enable the beef to soak in the garlic, ginger and Szechuan peppercorns as you slice it.

3. Lay the straightening iron steak on a baking sheet. Trim the beef into small slivers. Then toss the cornflour with the beef pieces.

4. Over the high fire, set a wok and add oils. Cautiously add in the beef strips and Szechuan chillies as the oil begins to burn.

5. Shift them around the wok quickly to stir-fry the meat on both sides.

6. Stir in the sauce until the beef is often cooked (4 minutes).

7. Enable it to boil and thicken the sauce.

8. Turn off the heat until it reaches the ideal consistency. Serve hot, seasoned with scallions and sesame seeds that are minced.

Chapter 5: Famous Keto Soups around the World

5.1 Italian Keto Soups and Broth Recipes

Italian Wedding Soup Keto and Low Carb

Cooking Time: 30 minutes

Serving Size: 6

Calories: 326

Ingredients:

- ½ cup (diced) carrots
- Salt and pepper to taste
- ½ cup almond flour
- 8 ounces raw spinach leaves (roughly chopped)
- ¼ cup fresh parsley (divided)
- 1 cup parmesan cheese grated
- 3 whole eggs
- 3 garlic cloves (grated)
- 2 tablespoons fresh basil
- ½ pound ground pork
- 10 cups chicken stock
- 3 cups cauliflower rice
- ½ pound ground beef

Method:

1. In a big pan, add the chicken stock and bring it to a simmer.

2. In a dish, add 1 egg, parsley, garlic, basil, almond flour, salt and pepper and blend. Add pork and beef (grounded) and combine when balanced, do not over-mix.

3. Shape the mini meatballs using a tiny scooper, then drop them into the boiling stock.

4. Simmer for ten minutes with the carrots and parmesan cheese rind.

5. Transfer the rice and spinach to the cauliflower, then finish cooking for another 7 minutes.

6. Shuffle the two remaining eggs and add them to the broth slowly, while the broth is stirring.

7. Heat for another few minutes and allow to cool gently with some grated parmesan cheese and a parsley garnish, before eating.

Italian Stracciatella Soup

Cooking Time: 10 minutes

Serving Size: 4

Calories: 151

Ingredients:

- 2 tablespoon (chopped) flat-leaf parsley
- sea salt and ground black pepper, to taste
- ⅛ teaspoon ground cinnamon
- 6 cups chicken stock or vegetable stock
- 4 tablespoon (grated) Parmesan cheese
- 2 large eggs

Method:

1. Slice the herbs and get all the ingredients ready.

2. In a big bowl, whisk the eggs gently, and then add the Parmesan cheese.

3. To a simmering boil, put the stock and cinnamon.

4. When simmering, stir in a clockwise direction, add the beaten eggs into the pot.

5. Turn heat off and enable the soup to sit before serving for a minute.

6. If needed, add pepper and salt to taste. Optionally, each bowl can be served with an extra tablespoon of fresh parsley and diced Parmesan cheese.

7. This soup is better eaten instantly, but can also be kept in the refrigerator and reheated within a day or two.

Italian Meatball Soup

Cooking Time: 35 minutes

Serving Size: 10

Calories: 111

Ingredients:

Meatballs:

- ¼ cup parmesan cheese
- ¼ cup almond flour
- 3 tablespoons white onion (grated)
- ½ pound ground beef
- 2 tablespoons egg (beaten)

- 3 tablespoons parsley (chopped)
- 1 clove garlic (minced)
- ½ teaspoon salt

Soup:

- 2 large eggs (beaten)
- 2 tablespoons parmesan cheese
- 2 cups baby spinach
- 10 cups chicken broth
- 1 cup cauliflower rice

Method:

1. In a middle-sized dish, combine all the meatball ingredients.
2. In your hands, shape heaping teaspoons of meatball paste into one inch shaped meatballs. On a broad cookie sheet, put the meatballs.
3. Move the chicken broth to a low simmer in a large soup pot.
4. While you add meatballs and cauliflower rice, lower the temperature and simmer.
5. Simmer for ten minutes or until the meatballs are thoroughly cooked. As the meatballs cook, the bubble will form, but it will subside as you boil the broth.
6. Add the fresh spinach and heat until softened, for two minutes.
7. Add the eggs and also the parmesan cheese in.
8. In a clockwise direction, stir and slowly pour the beaten eggs into the pot, stirring for two minutes with a fork until the strands are shaped.

9. Garnished with grated parmesan cheese for serving.

Keto Zuppa Toscana

Cooking Time: 45 minutes

Serving Size: 10

Calories: 247

Ingredients:

- 1 pound ground Italian sausage
- 1 tablespoon (minced) garlic
- 8 cups chicken broth
- ½ teaspoon (crushed) red pepper
- 6 slices bacon
- 5 cups spinach/coarsely (chopped)
- ½ teaspoon xanthan gum
- 4 cups cauliflower florets
- 1 cup heavy cream
- ½ medium onion (diced)

Method:

1. In a roasting pan over medium-high heat, cook the Italian sausage and red pepper flakes until crispy, golden brown, and no longer pink, for 15 minutes.

2. Remove from the pan, rinse, and put aside. The way is to break the sausage so that you do not fry it in the water.

3. Add the bacon, then fry until it is crispy. Remove the pan.

4. In the same roasting pan, add the garlic and onions; cook until the onions are soft and clear, for about five minutes.

5. Pour the chicken stock with the onion mixture into the roasting pan; bring it to a boil over high heat.

6. Insert the cauliflower and cook for about fifteen minutes, until the fork-tender.

7. Lower the heat to mild and stir in the fried sausage and the whipping cream; heat through.

8. A couple of minutes before eating, blend the spinach and bacon into the water.

9. Sprinkle the xanthan gum over the broth if you like a thicker broth, then quickly mix then boil until it thickens.

10. If required, you can cover it with grated Parmesan.

Italian Sausage Soup Instant Pot

Cooking Time: 45 minutes

Serving Size: 6

Calories: 294

Ingredients:

- 1 pound (ground) Italian sausage
- 2 cloves garlic crushed
- 32 ounces of beef broth (low-sodium)
- 4 ounces onion chopped
- 2 stalks celery chopped
- ½ teaspoon of sea salt

- basil (chopped) for garnish
- 2 ounces carrot diced
- ¼ teaspoon red pepper flakes
- 1 tablespoon fresh basil
- ¼ teaspoon (dried) oregano
- ¼ teaspoon black pepper (freshly ground)
- 15 ounces tomato sauce

Method:

1. In your Instant Cooker, put the inner pot.
2. To preheat the pot, pick the sauté option of your Instant Pot.
3. Add sausage if the word "cooked" appears on the screen.
4. Use the spoon to break down the bacon.
5. Brown, the sausage, stirring from time to time. Drain the excess fat from the pot if desired.
6. Stir in the onions, celery and carrot. Cook until they appear to settle, stirring periodically.
7. Add the beef broth, tomato sauce, garlic, basil, oregano, black pepper flakes of red pepper, and ½ teaspoon of sea salt to taste.
8. Cover the lid and lock it. In seal location, set steam release.
9. Pick the setting for the meat stew. You can change the time to thirty minutes using the +-keys.
10. Release the strain until the loop is already over. If needed, sprinkle a bit of fresh chopped parsley on top of each bowl.

Sausage Kale Soup

Cooking Time: 20 minutes

Serving Size: 8

Calories: 365

Ingredients:

- (shaved) Parmesan cheese
- 2 - 32-ounce chicken broth
- green onions
- ½ cup heavy cream
- salt and pepper, to taste
- 1 pound (ground) sweet Italian pork sausage
- 1 head cauliflower (chopped)
- 1 bunch red kale (removed and chopped)
- ¼ cup lemon juice
- 1 tablespoon (dried) oregano
- ½ cup (diced) onions
- 2 tablespoons minced garlic

Method:

1. In a big saucepan, sauté the sausage and onion until tender. Insert the garlic and cook a moment more.

2. To the pot, add the lemon juice, oregano, chicken broth and cauliflower. Get it to a low boil.

3. Reduce the flame and boil until the cauliflower is tender or for ten minutes.

4. Stir in the kale and the heavy cream and let it rest for five minutes until the kale wilts. Sprinkle with salt to taste.

5. Use shaved Parmesan cheese and spring onions to eat the spicy broth.

Low Carb Crock Pot Pizza Soup

Cooking Time: 8 hours 15 minutes

Serving Size: 8

Calories: 332

Ingredients:

- 1 cup (grated) mozzarella cheese
- ¼ cup (grated) parmesan cheese
- 1 can (crushed) tomatoes
- ½ lb. pepperoni (thinly sliced)
- 1 teaspoon garlic powder
- 1 small onion (diced)
- 1 lb. Italian sausage
- 2 cans beef broth
- 1 medium green pepper (diced)
- 2 teaspoons (dried) oregano
- 2 cans mushrooms
- 2 teaspoons Italian seasoning

Method:

1. Sauté until the sausage is golden.
2. Drain the sausage liquid and put it in a crockpot.
3. Add all the other items to the crockpot (excluding the cheeses).

4. Cook in a low, slow cooker for 6-8 hours.

5. Toss with cheese and pour into pots.

5.2 Winter Comfort Keto Soups Recipes

Keto Broccoli and Leek Soup Recipe

Cooking Time: 20 minutes

Serving Size: 5

Calories: 268

Ingredients:

- 1 teaspoon Pepper
- 1 tablespoon Parsley (chopped)
- 2 ½ cups chicken stock
- 1 teaspoon salt
- 1 medium Leek
- 1 pound Broccoli
- ½ cup Heavy Cream
- 1 clove garlic
- 3 ounces butter (salted)

Method:

1. Chop the white portion of the leek finely and put, along with the garlic and butter, in a wide saucepan.

2. Over low flame, sauté the leeks until they begin to become translucent. Put some milk.

3. Split the broccoli into florets of an exact size and put them in the saucepan.

4. Insert and stir the chicken broth. Make sure that it is mostly covered with broccoli.

5. Simmer for ten minutes over low to medium temperature. If the broccoli is cooked too soon, it can discolor and transform the soup dark.

6. When it is quick to disassemble with a spoon, the broccoli is ready.

7. Use a stick mixer to mix the soup gently, so there are no lumps left.

8. Use salt, pepper, and parsley to prepare. Change the spice according to taste.

Keto Cream of Mushroom Soup Recipe

Cooking Time: 40 minutes

Serving Size: 4

Calories: 439

Ingredients:

- 3 tablespoons tamari
- 3.5 ounces Butter
- 1 teaspoon Pepper
- 3 ounces Leek (sliced)
- 7 ounces Heavy Cream
- 1 pound mushrooms (quartered)
- 1 tablespoon butter (optional)
- 25 fluid ounces chicken stock
- 4 cloves garlic (roughly chopped)
- 4 ounces mushrooms (sliced)
- 1 pinch Salt (optional)

Method:

1. Place the butter, leek and garlic in a wide saucepan and sauté over moderate flame.

2. Insert the diced mushrooms and stir when the leek has warmed, and continue cooking for two minutes.

3. Transfer the chicken stock and tamari and boil for 20 minutes.

4. Add the cream and peppers and lift the saucepan from the flame.

5. Use a stick blender to mix until all ingredients are pureed.

6. When using the additional ingredients, over high heat, put the butter and salt in a non-stick frying pan.

7. Insert sliced mushrooms and sauté until cooked thoroughly, for 3 minutes.

8. Ladle the soup in bowls and garnish before eating it with the sautéed mushrooms.

Keto Taco Soup Recipe

Cooking Time: 25 minutes

Serving Size: 4

Calories: 201

Ingredients:

- 3 teaspoon Cilantro thinly (sliced)
- 3 tablespoon Sour Cream
- ½ cup Cheddar Cheese (grated)
- ½ medium Avocado (diced)
- 2 tablespoon butter
- 5 ounces Low Carb Pork Caritas

- 1 teaspoon Pepper
- ½ teaspoon Salt
- 1 medium green pepper (diced)
- 1 clove garlic (crushed)
- 8 ounces Tomato Puree
- 2 cups chicken stock
- 1 teaspoon (dried) oregano
- 1 teaspoon Cumin
- 1 teaspoon Paprika

Method:

1. Place the butter, sliced pepper and garlic in a medium saucepan and sauté for three minutes over a moderate flame until the butter is bubbling.

2. Insert the oregano, paprika and cumin and sauté until fragrant for another three minutes.

3. Add the chicken broth and tomatoes puree and get it to a simmer.

4. Transfer the caritas, salt and black pepper to the meat. Enable two minutes to cook to make sure the pork is cooked through.

5. Garnish the broth with sliced cheddar, chopped avocado, cilantro and sour cream in three bowls.

Keto Lamb Shanks Pressure Cooker Recipe

Cooking Time: 1 hour 15 minutes

Serving Size: 2

Calories: 588

Ingredients:

- 1 cup lamb broth
- 14 ounce (diced) tomatoes
- ¼ cup olive oil
- 1 teaspoon salt
- ½ teaspoon pepper
- 2.5 pounds lamb shanks
- 2 sticks celery (diced)
- 2 tablespoons Rosemary fresh
- 2 cloves garlic finely (chopped)
- 1 medium onion (diced)

Method:

1. Over a high flame, put your slow cooker and put half of the oil.
2. Dark the shanks and set it aside.
3. To the pressure cooker, transfer the remaining oil and add garlic, onions, celery and rosemary. Sauté when scented.
4. Combine the salt, pepper and lamb bread, blend properly, and then insert the diced tomatoes.
5. To the slow cooker, return the shanks and confirm that they are covered in the sauce.

6. Put the lid on the cooker and position it under high pressure. For fifty minutes, cook.

7. Turn off the temperature and allow fifteen minutes to rapid depressurization the cooker.

8. Open the cover and separate the shanks from the sauce, set it aside and cover to stay warm with foil.

9. To minimize the mixture, position the pressure cooker over medium temperature for ten minutes.

10. With a side of creamy Cauliflower Mash, serve the shanks.

Keto Beef Stroganoff Recipe

Cooking Time: 2 hours 15 minutes

Serving Size: 12

Calories: 482

Ingredients:

- 1 pound mushrooms (sliced)
- 1 cup sour cream
- ¼ cup olive oil
- ¼ cup red wine vinegar
- 2 cups beef stock
- 1 small onion (diced)
- 1 teaspoon pepper (ground)
- ¼ cup tomato paste
- 3 pounds Beef Brisket (thinly sliced)
- 1-2 teaspoons salt

- 2 cloves garlic (crushed)
- 2 teaspoons (Dried) thyme

Method:

1. Over a high flame, position a large saucepan. Add garlic, onion, thyme and oil.

2. Sauté until the onion starts to become visible. Insert the beef, salt and black pepper and sauté until golden brown.

3. Add the paste and cook the tomatoes for five minutes.

4. Insert the red wine vinegar and stir thoroughly. Leave five minutes of cooking.

5. Add the stock of beef and get it to a simmer. Simmer disclosed itself for 1 hour.

6. For another hour, add the mushrooms and begin to cook.

7. Take and stir in the sour cream from the flame.

8. If needed, test and add additional salt and black pepper.

9. Serve right away with the Buttery Cauliflower Mash on the side.

Homemade Corned Beef Soup with Low Carb Mustard Sauce

Cooking Time: 2 hours 15 minutes

Serving Size: 12

Calories: 441

Ingredients:

- 2 tablespoon salt
- 34 oz. Beef Stock
- 1 tablespoon whole peppercorns
- 3 cloves garlic (Cut in half)
- ¼ cup red wine vinegar
- 4.2 pound (Pickled) beef
- 2 tablespoon Lemon Thyme
- 1 Carrot Large Dice
- 2 tablespoon olive oil
- 1 Onion Large Dice

Low Carb Mustard Sauce

- 1 teaspoon pepper
- 1 pinch Salt
- 1.5 cup heavy cream
- 1 tablespoon parsley finely (chopped)
- 2.4 oz. Butter
- 2 tablespoon Dijon mustard

Method:

1. With a clean towel, rinsed the pickled beef thoroughly. Have your ingredients set.

2. Sauté the carrot, onion, garlic and thyme in olive oil for four minutes over the medium temperature in your slow cooker.

3. Insert the red wine vinegar, peppercorns, and salt and simmer for two minutes.

4. Add the beef and spill over the beef broth.

5. Based on the size of the beef and even the size of the slow cooker, you will need to add somewhat more water or less stock.

6. Bring the stock to a boil and firmly add the slow cooker lid to the bottom.

7. Continue cooking on high heat before steam is released from your pressure cooker, then reduce the heat to lower and allow to cook for two hours, or one hour per 1kg.

8. Turn off the heating after two hours and leave for twenty minutes to slowly relieve the pressure, then gently open the pressure valve on the lid to reduce any extra pressure and slide the cover off.

9. If you have a considerable portion, consider using a pair of tongs to grasp the meat from the top and a strong spoon or lifter under the bottom to hold the weight.

10. Immediately remove the corned beef. Cut the corned beef.

11. Since the contents of the pot are very salty, it can be strained and used to spice soups if you like, or discard the boiling liquid and veggies.

12. In a small skillet, mix the butter and mustard over a low flame.

13. Insert the milk and merge. The butter and the cream will remain separate initially but will come together as the heat increases.

14. Be very careful not to heat the sauce, so it is not going to mix. As the milk reduces the thickening of the sauce, you want the milk to be reduced by half.

15. To eat, insert the sliced parsley, salt and pepper, and drizzle over the corned beef.

Keto Lamb Stew Recipe

Cooking Time: 2 hours 20 minutes

Serving Size: 15

Calories: 462

Ingredients:

- 4 pounds lamb
- 1 onion large (dice)
- ¼ cup rosemary leaves
- ½ pound mushrooms (sliced)
- ½ cup tallow
- 1 cup tomato puree
- 1 teaspoon pepper
- ½ cup red wine vinegar
- 3 sticks celery
- 1 teaspoon salt
- 4 cups beef stock
- 3 cloves garlic (crushed)

Method:

1. At the bottom of your slow cooker, put the tallow, onion, garlic, rosemary and celery. For five minutes, sauté over moderate flame.

2. Add salt, the vinegar of red wine pepper, and puree of tomatoes. For another five minutes, keep cooking.

3. Add the stock of beef and mix well.

4. Place the lamb shoulder in the pot carefully, making sure the fluid just surrounds it. Until the lamb is filled, add additional beef stock or water.

5. Set the lid on the slow cooker and bring it to a boil. Switch the dial to the optimum pressure setting and allow pressurization to take place.

6. Drop the heat to low until your cooker starts releasing steam and leave to cook for 2 hours or 30 minutes per lb.

7. Remove the pressure cooker's cover and remove the slice of lamb's shoulder softly.

8. Return the pressure cooker to medium-high heat and allow the liquid to boil and decrease by ¼.

9. Using tongs to take the lamb meat off the bone as the liquid is diminishing and cut into bite-sized chunks approximately.

10. Return the chopped lamb beef, along with the mushrooms, to the pressure cooker and simmer for ten minutes.

11. Serve and eat two tablespoons of Sour Cream and add a tablespoon of Ribbed Parmesan Cheese.

5.3 Spicy Keto Soups and Broth Recipes

Keto Hot Chili Soup

Cooking Time: 30 minutes

Serving Size: 4

Calories: 369.5

Ingredients:

- 1 teaspoon coriander seeds
- Juice of half a lime
- Salt and pepper to taste
- 2 ounces queso fresco
- 4 tablespoons (chopped) fresh cilantro
- 2 tablespoons butter
- 1 medium avocado
- 2 tablespoons olive oil
- 4 tablespoons tomato paste
- 16 ounces chicken thighs
- 2 medium chilli peppers (sliced)
- 2 cups chicken broth
- 1 teaspoon turmeric
- ½ teaspoon ground cumin
- 2 cups of water

Method:

1. Break and put your chicken thighs in an oiled pan to prepare. Set it aside to rest until cooked.

2. In two tablespoons warm up the coriander seeds with olive oil to produce some of their aromas. Once it is fragrant, add the sliced chilli to the oil to season.

3. Add the broth and water to it and let it boil. Add seasonings.

4. Insert the tomato paste and butter and stir to melt and mix after simmering. For 10 minutes, let your soup boil.

5. Add the remaining the lime juice.

6. Into your bowls, place 4 ounces of chicken thighs and ladle the soup for serving. Garnish each bowl with ¼ avocado, half an ounce of fresh cheese, and cilantro.

Spicy Cauliflower Soup

Cooking Time: 20 minutes

Serving Size: 6

Calories: 251

Ingredients:

- ½ teaspoon of sea salt
- 1 medium spring onion
- 1 large cauliflower
- 1 medium Spanish chorizo sausage
- 3 tablespoon ghee
- 1 medium turnip
- 2 cups vegetable stock
- 1 small white onion (chopped)

Method:

1. Clean and dice the cauliflower into tiny florets.

2. Grease 2 teaspoons of ghee in a big soup pot or a Dutch oven and add the chopped onion. Cook until finely browned on a medium-high flame.

3. When stirring, add the cauliflower and cook for about five minutes. Use the cap to add the chicken broth and cover.

4. Cook and turn off the heat for about ten minutes.

5. Dice the sausage with chorizo. Peel and dice the turnip finely or use more cauliflower-for browning, the stems are great.

6. Place the remainder ghee on a heavy-based skillet and cook over medium-high heat until the chorizo is golden and the turnip is around 10 minutes ready.

7. Shift half of the blend of chorizo and turnip into the soup. Stir until thick and creamy with the use of a hand blender.

8. Season with cayenne pepper and salt. Optionally, 1 cup of heavy whipping cream can be added.

Spicy Low Carb Hamburger Soup

Cooking Time: 25 minutes

Serving Size: 14

Calories: 278

Ingredients:

- 1 medium ripe avocado (peeled and seeded)
- 3 cups (pre-shredded) Mexican Style cheese blend
- 1 can (sliced) pickled jalapenos

- 1 can pure pumpkin
- ¾ cups (chopped) celery
- ½ teaspoon table salt
- 2 lbs. ground beef chuck
- 8 cups beef broth
- ½ teaspoon onion powder
- ½ teaspoon ground cayenne pepper
- 1 tablespoon ground cumin
- ¾ teaspoon granulated garlic
- 1 tablespoon chilli powder
- 1 tablespoon smoked paprika

Method:

1. Combine the chilli powder, garlic, paprika, onion powder, cumin, cayenne and salt in a shallow cup. Just put aside.

2. Brown ground beef in a large roasting pan until almost completed and add previously made seasoning mixture, stirring to integrate into the meat fully.

3. Insert the celery and continue sautéing for about two more minutes. Place the beef broth in it and get it to a boil.

4. Meanwhile, puree the pumpkin, jalapenos and avocado in a blender until creamy.

5. To the boiling fluid, add the puree and stir until completely incorporated and smooth. Turn the heat off. Stir the cheese in.

6. Garnish with more fruit, cheese and your favourite hot sauce for each mug.

Low Carb Spicy Chicken Soup

Cooking Time: 30 minutes

Serving Size: 4

Calories: 405

Ingredients:

- 1 tablespoon chicken bouillon paste
- 1 teaspoon turmeric
- 10 ounces canned tomato and chillies
- 1 onion (chopped)
- 0.5 cup full-fat coconut milk
- 6 cloves garlic
- 2 julienned ginger

For the Chicken

- 2 cups Swiss chard (chopped)
- 1.5 cups (chopped) celery
- 1 pound Boneless Skinless Chicken Thighs

For Finishing

- ½ cup Full-Fat Coconut Milk

Method:

1. In a blender, combine the onion, ginger, garlic, tomatoes and chillies, turmeric, broth base, and coconut milk, and whisk until the sauce is roughly pureed.

2. Pour the mixture into your quick pot's internal liner. Add chopped meat, Swiss chard and sliced celery to the mix.

3. Cook the soup for five minutes on increased speed and allow it to relieve pressure for ten minutes naturally. Release all the weight left.

4. Stir in the leftover ½ cup coconut milk, mix and serve.

30 Minute Spicy Keto Ramen Bowl

Cooking Time: 30 minutes

Serving Size: 5

Calories: 103

Ingredients:

- 3 packets shirataki noodles
- 5 cups bone broth
- 1 tablespoon oil
- 4 oz. mushrooms (sliced thin)
- 4 hard-boiled eggs
- ¼ cup of soy sauce
- ¼ cup rice wine vinegar
- 1 onion (sliced)
- ¼ teaspoon pepper
- 1 tablespoon fish sauce
- 1 tablespoon ginger
- ½ teaspoon salt
- 3 cloves garlic
- 1 teaspoon chilli paste

Method:

1. Add oil and cook under moderate heat in a large soup pot. Sauté the onions until tender, for 3 minutes.

2. Add the rest of the ingredients (excluding noodles and egg) to the cup. For 20-30 minutes, boil under low-medium pressure.

3. Take the noodles from the bag, and clean under cold water very well.

4. Change the broth's seasoning. Stir the noodles in.

5. Divide the broth into bowls and portions. If needed, add cut boiled eggs, sliced beef or chicken, cilantro, sesame seeds, sliced green onion and additional chilli.

Keto Spicy Chicken Pozole

Cooking Time: 50 minutes

Serving Size: 6

Calories: 215

Ingredients:

- Chicken breast boneless skinless 1-¼ pound
- Water 3 cup
- Coarse kosher salt 2 teaspoon
- Avocado oil 1-½ tablespoon
- Chile 8 gram
- Dried guajillo chilli pepper 5 grams
- Boiling water 1-½ cup
- Cilantro ½ cup (chopped)
- Cabbage green 2 cup

- Radish 8 small
- Avocado 1 each
- Garlic, fresh 3 clove
- Chicken broth 30 ounce

Method:

1. Destem the chillies in a blender jug. Add 1½ cups of boiling water to the mixture.

2. Use a spoon to drag the chillies down into the warm water. Enable 10-15 minutes to rehydrate the chillies.

3. Over medium heat, heat a six-quart sauté pan until hot. Insert the avocado oil to the pan and swirl.

4. Insert a chopped breast of chicken. Sauté for 4 minutes on the first side before brown, then stir in the meat and brown at the other side.

5. With a quarter of the salt, season.

6. Add the cloves of garlic to the washed chillies and use a food processor to puree everything.

7. In the roasting pan, add the chicken broth and the chilli puree. Add a little bit of chilli puree at a time and check after the chicken is fried, if you do not want a lot of moisture.

8. Add more as needed. Bring the broth to a boil and simmer until the chicken is soft, or for thirty minutes.

9. Season the other portion of the salt with the broth.

10. Chop the cabbage thinly, slice the radishes thinly, chop the cilantro and chop the avocado to prepare the toppings.

Low Carb Chicken Fajita Soup

Cooking Time: 3 hours 20 minutes

Serving Size: 8

Calories: 306

Ingredients:

- 2 lbs. boneless skinless chicken breasts
- 2½ tablespoon homemade taco seasoning
- salt and pepper to taste
- 2½ cups chicken broth
- ½ cup heavy whipping cream
- 1 cup chicken broth
- 6 oz. cream cheese
- 2 10 oz. cans (diced) tomatoes with green chillies
- 1 onion (chopped)
- 1 tablespoon butter
- 1 green pepper (chopped)
- 3 garlic cloves (minced)

Method:

1. In a slow cooker, prepare the boneless skinless chicken thighs for three hours on high, or six hours on low in a chicken broth cup. Season with pepper/salt.

2. Remove from the slow cooker and slice when the chicken is finished. (The remaining broth for the soup must be strainer).

3. Sauté the green pepper, tomato, and garlic in one tablespoon of butter in a wide saucepan until they are translucent.

4. Mash the cream cheese onto the vegetables with a spoon so that it can smoothly mix as it melts.

5. Connect the chicken broth, dried tomatoes, healthy whipping cream, and taco seasoning.

6. Simmer on low for twenty minutes uncovered.

7. For ten minutes, add shredded chicken and simmer. To taste, add salt and black pepper.

8. Optional: Use grated cheese, coriander, spring onions, avocado, and sour cream to top each cup.

5.4 Famous Keto Soups in the World

Keto Broccoli Cheddar Soup

Cooking Time: 40 minutes

Serving Size: 6

Calories: 512

Ingredients:

- 6 oz. cream cheese
- 4 cups (freshly grated) sharp cheddar
- 4 tablespoon (unsalted) butter
- 4 cups (low-sodium) chicken stock
- 6 cups small broccoli florets
- 1 large carrot (cut into matchsticks)
- Kosher salt
- (Freshly ground) black pepper
- 2 little cloves garlic, (minced)
- ¾ teaspoon ground mustard
- ¾ teaspoon onion powder
- ¾ teaspoon (smoked) paprika
- Pinch cayenne pepper

Method:

1. Melt the butter in a medium saucepan.
2. Add the garlic and carrot and simmer for about two minutes, stirring until it is fragrant.
3. Stir in paprika, powdered mustard, onion powder, and cayenne.

4. Load the chicken stock into the mixture and get it to a boil. Season with pepper and salt.

5. Insert the broccoli and cook for around 5 minutes, until tender.

6. Add the cheese and cheddar cheese and cook, stirring, until molten.

7. Season with pepper and salt and serve hot.

Roasted Butternut Squash Soup

Cooking Time: 40 minutes

Serving Size: 4

Calories: 377

Ingredients:

- 1 tablespoon fresh thyme
- 1 quarter (low-sodium) chicken broth
- 1 large butternut squash (peeled and cubed)
- (Freshly ground) black pepper
- 1 stalk celery (thinly sliced)
- 1 large carrot (chopped)
- 1 tablespoon butter
- 1 onion (chopped)
- 2 potatoes (peeled and chopped)
- 3 tablespoon (extra-virgin) olive oil
- Kosher salt

Method:

1. Preheat the oven to 400 degrees.

2. Toss the butternut squash and potato with two tablespoons of olive oil on a wide baking sheet and sprinkle generously with pepper and salt.

3. For twenty-five minutes, roast until crispy.

4. In the meantime, over a moderate flame, melt the butter and the remaining tablespoon of olive oil in a big pot.

5. Add the onion, carrots, and celery and simmer for 10 to 15 minutes, until tender.

6. With pepper, salt, and thyme, season generously.

7. Pour over the chicken broth and add the roasted squash and potatoes.

8. Simmer for ten minutes, then mix the soup until smooth, using an electric mixer. (Alternatively, pass batches of hot broth carefully to a food processor.)

9. Spiced with thyme, serve.

Keto Chili Soup

Cooking Time: 45 minutes

Serving Size: 8

Calories: 324

Ingredients:

- (Sliced) green onions
- (Sliced) avocado
- 2 celery stalks (chopped)
- 2 cups (low-sodium) beef broth
- Sour cream (for garnish)

- 2 teaspoon (dried) oregano
- 2 tablespoon smoked paprika
- 2 cloves garlic (minced)
- 2 teaspoon ground cumin
- Kosher salt
- 1 green bell pepper (chopped)
- ½ cups sliced baby Bella's
- (Freshly ground) black pepper
- 3 slices bacon (cut into ½ strips)
- ¼ medium yellow onion (chopped)
- 2 lb. ground beef
- 2 tablespoon chilli powder
- (Shredded) cheddar

Method:

1. Cook the bacon in a big pot over medium heat. Pick the bacon from the pot with a slotted spoon until it is crisp.

2. Transfer the onion, pepper, and mushrooms to the pot and simmer for 5 minutes, until tender.

3. Include the garlic and cook until fragrant, for an additional 1 minute.

4. Move the vegetables and transfer the beef to one side of the plate. Cook, stirring regularly until there is no remaining pink.

5. Drain the fat and place back to the heat. Season with salt and add chilli powder, cilantro, oregano, and paprika.

6. Stir to mix and simmer for an additional two minutes. Stir in the broth and get it to a boil.

7. Let it cook for another five to ten minutes until much of the broth has evaporated.

8. Cover with sour cream, reserved pork, cheese, spring onions, and avocado and put in cups.

Cream of Asparagus Soup

Cooking Time: 40 minutes

Serving Size: 4

Calories: 425

Ingredients:

- (Freshly chopped) chives
- (Freshly chopped) dill
- 2 tablespoon butter
- 2 cups (low-sodium) chicken broth
- ½ cups heavy cream
- 1 clove garlic (minced)
- Freshly ground black pepper
- 2 lb. asparagus (trimmed)
- Kosher salt

Method:

1. Melt some butter in a large pot over medium heat.

2. Add the garlic and roast for two minutes until it is fragrant.

3. Include the asparagus, sprinkle with salt, and simmer for five minutes, until golden.

4. Add liquid and boil, covered, until asparagus is very crispy but still green, 15 to 20 minutes.

5. Purée broth, using an immersion or standard blender.

6. To prevent overheating the broth, make sure to pause and remove the lid a couple of times if you have a standard blender.

7. Put it back in the jar, stir in the cream, and then warm over medium heat. To taste, season with pepper and salt.

8. Garnish with more spices and cream.

Chicken Avocado Lime Soup

Cooking Time: 35 minutes

Serving Size: 6

Calories: 373

Ingredients:

- 3 tablespoon fresh lime juice
- 3 medium avocados (peeled and diced)
- 1 ½ lb. boneless skinless chicken breasts
- Salt and (freshly ground) black pepper
- ¼ cup (chopped) cilantro
- 2 Roma tomatoes (seeded and diced)
- ½ teaspoon ground cumin
- 3 cloves garlic (minced)
- 4 cans (low-sodium) chicken broth
- 1 tablespoon olive oil

- 1 ¼ cups (chopped) green onions
- 2 jalapeños (seeded and minced)

Method:

1. Heat one tablespoon of olive oil over the moderate flame in a big pot.

2. Once the onion and jalapenos are warm, add the spring onions and sauté until soft, about two minutes, adding the garlic for the last 30 seconds.

3. Add chicken broth, onions, cumin, add salt and pepper to taste and, if used, add chicken breasts.

4. Bring the mixture over medium-high heat to a boil.

5. Then reduce heat to moderate, cover with the lid and enable to cook, occasionally stirring, until the chicken has cooked for 15 minutes (cooking time can vary depending on chicken breast thickness).

6. Lower the burner to warm fire, move the chicken from the pan and leave for five minutes to sit on a cutting board, then slice the chicken and transfer to the broth.

7. Stir in coriander and lime juice, and, if used, rotisserie chicken.

8. Transfer the avocados to the soup just before serving.

Greek Lemon Chicken Soup

Cooking Time: 30 minutes

Serving Size: 2

Calories: 214

Ingredients:

- ¼ cup (chopped) chive
- Salt and pepper
- 10 cups chicken broth
- ½ teaspoons (crushed) red pepper
- 2 ounces (crumbled) feta
- 2 boneless skinless chicken breasts
- 1 cup Israeli couscous (pearl)
- 1 sweet onion
- 1 large lemon (zested)
- 3 tablespoon olive oil
- 8 cloves garlic (minced)

Method:

1. Put the coconut oil over medium-low heat in a wide saucepot.
2. Just peel the onion. Half it, then cut it into small slices.
3. Sauté the onions and the minced garlic for 4 minutes to loosen until the oil is heated.
4. Transfer to the pot the chicken broth, raw chicken thighs, lime juice and crushed red pepper.
5. Boost the heat, cover it, and bring it to a boil.
6. Decrease the heat to mild after boiling, then simmer for five minutes.

7. Stir in 1 teaspoon of salt and black pepper to taste. Simmer for 5 more minutes. Switch off the heat then.

8. Take the two chicken thighs out of the pot using tweezers.

9. To slice the chicken, use a spoon and tweezers.

10. Place it down to a simmer then. Stir in the crumbled chives and sliced feta cheese.

11. Season with salt and pepper as needed. Serve it warm.

Skinny Buffalo Chicken Soup

Cooking Time: 45 minutes

Serving Size: 8

Calories: 236

Ingredients:

- 1 cup Buffalo Sauce
- (Chopped) green onion and blue cheese
- 2 pounds rotisserie chicken (cooked and shredded)
- 1 medium onion (diced)
- 1 tablespoon butter
- 1 pound (sliced) carrots
- 6 stalks of celery (sliced)
- 2 cups chicken broth
- 1 cup of water
- 3 tablespoon ranch seasoning
- 1 large head of cauliflower (chopped)

- 4 cups chicken stock

Method:

1. In the stockpot, cook cauliflower in water, ranch dressing, chicken stock, and chicken broth until very tender; about ten minutes.

2. Sauté the celery, carrots, and onion with the butter while the cauliflower is frying.

3. Till the onions are transparent and the veggies are fork ready, cook on medium-high heat.

4. In the slow cooker, mix the cauliflower into a puree using an electric mixer.

5. It should be thoroughly blended, and the broth should form a thicker foundation. Insert and whisk in the hot sauce.

6. To the stockpot, add the celery, garlic, and onions and stir.

7. Stir in the chicken and allow to cook for 30 minutes on low flame.

8. Serve warm as a garnish of spring onion and blue cheese.

Instant Pot Philly Cheesesteak Soup Recipe

Cooking Time: 50 minutes

Serving Size: 8

Calories: 259

Ingredients:

- 2 hoagie rolls (sliced)
- 8 slices provolone cheese
- 1 ½ lb. shaved beef
- 8 ounces cremini mushrooms (sliced)
- 4 cups beef broth
- ¼ cup Worcestershire sauce
- 3 medium sweet onions (thinly sliced)
- 2 green bell peppers (thinly sliced)
- 2 tablespoons of liquid smoke
- kosher salt and black pepper
- 1 tablespoon (unsalted) butter
- 2 tablespoons olive oil

Method:

1. Place the beef in a big pan.
2. Transfer the sauce, liquid smoke, salt, and pepper to the Worcestershire.
3. Blend and mix. Enable the beef to marinate while you prepare the veggies at low temperatures.
4. Set to sauté the slow cooker. Add the butter and coconut oil.

5. Add the onions as the butter is melted. With pepper and salt, season.

6. Cook, stirring regularly for about ten minutes or until the onions are soft and approximately half the volume has been reduced.

7. Add the peppers and mushrooms and cook until the vegetables are tender, for an extra 5 minutes.

8. Add seasoned beef from the bottom of the pan to the Instant Pot and any accumulated fluids. Stir to combine. Pour the broth down.

9. Place the lid on the instant pot and cook for twenty minutes under high pressure. Enable the soup to depressurize spontaneously.

10. Break rolls of hoagie into 1 inch thick strips.

11. Place under the broiler on a cookie sheet and toast for around 2 minutes on either side. To stop flames, watch closely.

12. Ladle the soup into healthy oven cups. Add 1 or 2 slices of toast and 1 slice of Provolone cheese to each cup.

13. Place the bowls on a baking tray and place for around 60 seconds under the broiler or until the cheese is melted. Immediately serve.

Chapter 6: Asian Ketogenic Vegetarian Recipes

This chapter will cover all tasty and delicious recipes of vegetarian meals including breakfast recipes, lunch recipes, dinner recipes, soups and side dish recipes.

6.1 Keto Vegetarian Recipes for Breakfast

Keto Coconut Flake Pancakes Recipe

Cooking Time: 15 minutes

Serving Size: 2

Calories: 238

Ingredients:

- 2 eggs
- 3 tablespoon coconut flour
- ½ tablespoon vanilla essence (optional)
- pinch of salt (optional)
- 2 tablespoon thickened cream
- 1 tablespoon melted butter
- 1 tablespoon sweetener
- ½ tablespoon baking powder

Method:

1. Beat the eggs together with a touch of salt in a medium-sized dish.
2. Put together all the coconut flour, baking flour and the flavouring in another dish.

3. To combine the ingredients, add softened butter, thickened cream and vanilla essence.

4. Integrate the dry products and blend them all into the wet ones.

5. Let the combination rest for at least ten minutes before tiny air bubbles begin to form on top, allowing the pancake mix to thicken up as well.

6. Over the low-medium fire, steam a pan and spray with butter or avocado oil.

7. Pour roughly ¼ cup of flour on the pan per pancakes. Fry the nut flour pancakes on either side for 2 minutes and set aside until they are fried.

Breakfast Feta and Veggie Egg Muffins

Cooking Time: 15 minutes

Serving Size: 12

Calories: 321

Ingredients:

- ½ cup feta cheese
- Parmesan for topping
- 12 eggs
- 1 pack spinach
- ¼ jalapeno (chopped)
- ¼ cup almond milk
- 7 mushrooms
- 1 tablespoon turmeric

- ¼ tablespoon salt
- Pepper to taste
- ½ tablespoon baking powder
- 1.5 tablespoon garlic powder
- ½ tablespoon onion powder

Method:

1. Heat the oven to 350.
2. Mix the eggs, milk and spices in a large dish.
3. Whisk when they're mixed.
4. Chop and add the vegetables to the dish.
5. Whisk until they are mixed.
6. Blend with the feta.
7. Spray non-stick moisturizer on a muffin tray and part the mix into the cups. Use parmesan to brush the edges.
8. Bake for fifteen minutes, turn the pan over and cook for 14 more minutes.
9. Let the pan sit until its cold.

Keto Mixed Berry Smoothie Recipe

Cooking Time: 3 minutes

Serving Size: 1

Calories: 254

Ingredients:

- 1 teaspoon sweetener
- 3 cubes of ice

- ¼ cup of coconut milk
- ¼ cup of frozen mixed berries

Method:

1. In your blender, bring all the ingredients and whisk away for about one minute until it is creamy and well blended.

2. Instantly serve.

Decadent Low Carb Avocado Toast

Cooking Time: 25 minutes

Serving Size: 8

Calories: 318

Ingredients:

- 1 tablespoon seasoning salt
- 1 ½ cup almond flour
- 1 egg
- 4 ripe avocados
- 4 tablespoon fresh lemon juice
- 1 tablespoon olive oil
- ¾ tablespoon fresh oregano
- ¼ tablespoon crushed red pepper
- ½ tablespoon stevia
- ¼ cup of water
- ½ cup grated Parmesan cheese
- ½ tablespoon baking powder

Method:

1. Preheat oven to the 375.

2. In a small cup, mix the eggs, essential oil, and water.

3. Combine the almond flour, cheese, baking soda, and oregano, stevia, and red pepper flakes in a wide bowl and stir to balance.

4. To the flour mixture, add egg mixture and stir to form a sticky dough.

5. Cover a half pan sheet with a spray of olive oil and smooth the dough into a rectangle.

6. Bake for 25 minutes, until the sides are crispy and golden. Let the toast cool for about twenty minutes.

7. Organize the avocados, whereas the dough is cooling.

8. Put the avocados in a wide bowl with the lime juice and salt and mash well.

9. Slice six squares of the toast and finish with avocado. Instantly serve!

Keto Frappuccino Recipe

Cooking Time: 2 minutes

Serving Size: 1

Calories: 122

Ingredients:

- ¼ tablespoon Xanthan Gum

- 1 cup ice

- ½ cup strong brewed coffee (chilled)

- 2 tablespoon heavy cream

- 1 tablespoon sweetener
- ¼ cup (unsweetened) almond milk

Method:

1. In your blender, bring all the items and blend until smooth and mixed. (Approximately 1 minute)
2. Pour in a bowl or a cup and finish with any whipped cream that is keto-friendly and some other side dishes you want.

Veggie Scrambled Eggs

Cooking Time: 20 minutes

Serving Size: 2

Calories: 409

Ingredients:

- 1 tablespoon cayenne pepper
- ½ tablespoon salt
- 4 eggs
- 1 tablespoon bouillon powder
- ½ tablespoon turmeric powder
- 4 mini bell peppers
- ¼ red onions
- ¼ cup olive oil
- 1 tablespoon coconut milk

Method:

1. Chop the bell peppers and onions into medium-sized bits.

2. In a separate dish, split up the shells, add the coconut milk and salts and mix.

3. On medium-high heat, transfer olive oil to a pan and, when hot, add the grated onion and stir for two minutes.

4. Add the mini bell peppers, turmeric, bouillon powder, and cayenne pepper and mix over medium heat for five minutes.

5. Stir in the eggs, keep for about a minute, and then use a fork or a large serving spoon to break them apart.

6. After 2 minutes, remove it from the heat. Serve hot.

6.2 Keto Vegetarian Recipes for Lunch and Dinner

Vegan Arugula Avocado Tomato Salad

Cooking Time: 20 minutes

Serving Size: 8

Calories: 134

Ingredients:

Arugula Salad

- 2 large avocados
- ½ cup red onion (minced)
- 1-pint tomatoes (sliced)
- 1-pint red grape tomatoes (sliced)
- 5 oz. baby arugula (roughly chopped)
- 6 large basil leaves (thinly sliced)

Balsamic Vinaigrette

- ¼ tablespoon Himalayan pink sea salt
- ¼ tablespoon black pepper
- 2 tablespoon balsamic vinegar
- 1 tablespoon lemon juice
- 1 small garlic clove (minced)
- 1 tablespoon olive oil
- 1 tablespoon maple syrup

Method:

1. In a wide mixing cup, placed the finely chopped arugula and cut basil leaves.

2. Transfer to the cup the grape tomatoes, slices of avocado, and diced red onion.

3. Stir together 2 tablespoons of balsamic vinegar, 1 teaspoon of olive oil, 1 tablespoon of maple syrup, 1 tablespoon of lemon juice, 1 clove of garlic, ¼ teaspoon of cinnamon, and ¼ teaspoon of black pepper in a medium bowl until well mixed.

4. Over the salad, pour the balsamic sauce. Mix the salad carefully until the dressing is uniformly spread, then move the salad to a large bowl.

Paleo Triple Green Kale Salad

Cooking Time: 15 minutes

Serving Size: 4

Calories: 135

Ingredients:

Part 1 -

- 1 tablespoon grated fresh ginger
- Pinch of coarse sea salt
- 2 tablespoon (extra-virgin) olive oil
- 2 small garlic cloves
- 8-10 oz. kale
- 2 tablespoons toasted sesame oil

Part 2 -

- Orange zest
- Sprinkle with hemp seeds

- 1 ripe avocado (sliced)
- Scallions (chopped)
- 2 teaspoon balsamic vinegar
- Snow peas (chopped)
- 2 teaspoon coconut amino

Method:

1. Wash and carefully clean the kale.
2. On a chopping board, place a kale leaf and cut all the ends.
3. Stack and roll 5 levels of kale leave to chop into tiny chunks.
4. Mix all of the ingredients under 'Part 1' with sliced kale leaves.
5. Massage the kale softly with clean palms, pressing the oil onto the leaves for a few seconds.
6. Add ingredients to "Step 2", and give it a short toss.
7. Serve at ambient temperature or moderately chilled.

Tomato Mushroom Spaghetti Squash

Cooking Time: 40 minutes

Serving Size: 6

Calories: 173

Ingredients:

- Pinch of red pepper flakes (if desired)
- Optional: Parmesan cheese
- 1 large spaghetti squash

- 3 tablespoons olive oil
- ¼ cup onions or shallots (chopped)
- Kosher salt and black pepper
- 2 cups tomatoes (diced)
- ¼ cup pine nuts (toasted)
- fresh basil (a handful)
- 4 cloves garlic (minced)
- 8 ounces mushrooms (sliced)

Method:

1. Cook the squash spaghetti. Slice in two when cool enough to manage, cut seeds and shred them with two forks. Set the squash aside.

2. Heat the oil over moderate heat in a large sauté pan.

3. Add the mushrooms and onions, stirring continuously for about 4 minutes.

4. Add the garlic, then stir for another couple of minutes, until the garlic is fragrant. Do not brown the garlic.

5. Insert the tomatoes, and begin to stir.

6. Remove the cooked spaghetti squash and blend until the squash is hot and the vegetables are spread evenly.

7. Using new basil and toasted nuts to mix. When needed, season with kosher salt, pepper and a handful of red pepper flakes to satisfy.

Vegan Sesame Ginger Coleslaw

Cooking Time: 30 minutes

Serving Size: 12

Calories: 66

Ingredients:

Sesame Ginger Dressing

- 1 medium garlic clove (peeled)
- 2-inch knob fresh ginger (peeled)
- 1 tablespoon hot sauce
- 1 tablespoon maple syrup
- 2 tablespoon almond butter
- 2 tablespoon rice vinegar
- 3 tablespoon lime juice
- 1 tablespoon tahini
- 2 tablespoon (low-sodium) tamari

Coleslaw -

- 1 cup cilantro roughly (chopped)
- 1 cup green onions (sliced)
- 2 cups carrots (thinly sliced)
- 5 cups red cabbage (thinly sliced)
- 5 cups green cabbage (thinly sliced)

Method:

1. Place two tablespoons of almond butter, one tablespoon of tahini, two tablespoons of tamari, two tablespoons of rice vinegar, three tablespoons of lime juice, one tablespoon of hot sauce, one tablespoon of

maple syrup, one clove of garlic, and a 2-inch knob of ginger in a wide mixing bowl and combine until smooth and fluffy.

2. In a wide mixing cup, place the finely diced green and red cabbage, carrots, spring onions, and cilantro.

3. To blend, pour the seasoning over the cabbage mix and toss.

4. Before eating, seal and put the coleslaw in the fridge to cool for one hour.

Paleo Broccoli Fried Rice

Cooking Time: 8 minutes

Serving Size: 4

Calories: 87

Ingredients:

- 4 tablespoon (chopped) cilantro or parsley
- Sprinkle with (sliced) almonds
- 4 cups (riced) broccoli
- Quarter lime juice
- 2 bulbs scallions (chopped)
- ¼ coarse salt
- ¼ - ½ tablespoon (grated frozen) ginger
- 1 tablespoon coconut amino
- 1.5 tablespoon toasted sesame oil
- 1 tablespoon avocado oil
- 1 tablespoon (finely chopped) garlic

Method:

1. Add one tablespoon of ghee to a well-heated pan.

2. Sauté the riced broccoli for one min with roughly sliced garlic.

3. Add coconut amino, toasted sesame oil and coarse salt to spice the riced broccoli.

4. Sauté for an extra two minutes. Broccoli must be prepared with a certain crunch and not mushy until the colour is dark green.

5. Turn off the heating and grate about ½ teaspoon of frozen ginger over the rice whilst the broccoli rice is still high.

6. Add spring onions, cilantro, and diced almonds to garnish. Serve with the side of additional lime wedges.

6.3 Keto Vegetarian Soups and Sides

Lemon Garlic Oven Roasted Asparagus

Cooking Time: 22 minutes

Serving Size: 4

Calories: 67

Ingredients:

- 1 tablespoon fresh lemon juice
- 1tablespoon vegan parmesan cheese
- 1 lb. asparagus
- 2 garlic cloves (minced)
- 1 teaspoon olive oil
- salt and pepper
- ¼ teaspoon onion granules
- 1 teaspoon lemon zest
- 5 lemon slices
- 1 tablespoon olive oil
- ¼ tablespoon dried thyme

Method:

1. The oven should be preheated to 425 degrees.

2. Prepare the Asparagus: Rinse and clean the asparagus well enough.

3. You can either split the asparagus in two or let it snap spontaneously, or you can break off the base of the stalk by 1½ inches.

4. Season and Bake: Use a baking paper-lined tray to lay the asparagus spears.

5. Sprinkle over the asparagus with one tablespoon olive oil and toss to cover each slice.

6. Sprinkle generously over the asparagus with thyme, onion granules, lime juice, sea salt, and pepper and mix one more time. Use lemon wedges to the top and bake for eight minutes.

7. Mince the cloves of garlic and place them in a little bowl. Insert 1 teaspoon of olive oil and blend.

8. Remove the dish from the oven after cooking the asparagus and scatter the minced garlic uniformly over the tray.

9. Place the tray back in the oven and bake for an extra 4 minutes. Serve hot.

Low-Carb Roasted Cabbage with Lemon

Cooking Time: 35 minutes

Serving Size: 4

Calories: 78

Ingredients:

- 1 large head of green cabbage
- black pepper and salt
- 3 tablespoons lemon juice
- lemon slices
- 2 tablespoons olive oil

Method:

1. Preheat oven to 450F.
2. Use non-stick spray or olive oil to spray a baking dish.

3. Split the cabbage heads into eight wedges of the same length, cutting across the center and stem end.

4. Organize the roasting pan with wedges in a single sheet.

5. Mix the lime juice and olive oil.

6. Then spray the top sides of each cabbage slice with the combination using a large spoon and season with salt and pepper.

7. Then, gently turn the cabbage wedges, spray the second side with the combination of olive oil/lemon juice and season with salt and pepper.

8. Roast cabbage for about fifteen minutes, or until it is perfectly browned on the side that hits the pan.

9. Remove the pan from the heat, then gently turn each wedge.

10. Put back in the oven and roast for 15 more minutes, until the cabbage is well golden brown and cooked through with any residual chewiness.

Lamb and Herb Bone Broth

Cooking Time: 12 hours

Serving Size: 4

Calories: 52

Ingredients:

- 1-3 gallons of water
- Salt optional
- 1 pound lamb bones

- 3 sprigs Rosemary

- 3 sticks celery (roughly chopped)

- 3 cloves garlic

- 5 sprigs thyme

- 3 medium carrots

- 1 tablespoon olive oil

- 1 small onion large (diced)

Method:

1. Preheat oven at 390F.

2. Place the lamb bones in a grilling pan and cook until golden brown, for 40 minutes.

3. Insert the oil and position over moderate heat in a large slow cooker.

4. Insert the cabbage, carrot, celery, garlic, rosemary and thyme, and sauté for five minutes.

5. Insert the lamb bones and scrape into the pot with any fat or juices from the stockpot.

6. Add one gallon of water and allow to boil until the heat is reduced to a minimum.

7. Boil for 8-24 hours covered.

8. The amount of water that you need depends on how long you want the broth to boil for.

9. Strain the broth into a fine mesh strainer after the broth is boiled for the desired amount of time. Eat warm.

Chicken Feet Bone Broth

Cooking Time: 12 hours

Serving Size: 8

Calories: 104

Ingredients:

- 1 sprig of rosemary
- 4 quarts (filtered) water
- One ½ inch piece of fresh ginger
- 1 teaspoon salt
- 2 tablespoons apple cider vinegar
- 12 pastured chicken feet

Method:

1. Add the chicken feet and apple cider vinegar to a slow cooker and fill it with water until the feet are coated.
2. Get it to a boil, then cook for ten minutes. In cold water, squeeze and blanch the feet, enabling them to cool, then take the membranes off.
3. In a stockpot, add chicken feet.
4. Until the feet are coated, insert filtered water and bring it to a boil.
5. Add seasonings. Allow for twelve or more hours to boil on low heat.
6. Remove the water from the bone broth and allow it to cool.
7. Strain the liquid into plastic containers and serve or ice in the refrigerator instantly.

Conclusion

Increased-fats, modest-proteins, and quite-low-carbohydrates are mainly part of a ketogenic diet. The revival of the ketogenic diet as a formula for accelerated weight loss is a relatively recent phenomenon that, at least in the short term, has proved to be very successful. A relatively low-carbohydrates, high-fat diet that has specific links to the Atkins and low-carbohydrates diets is the ketogenic diet. It requires significantly lowering and replacing the intake of carbohydrates with fat. This carbohydrate reduction places the body in a metabolic condition called ketosis. For those that are overweight, obese or looking to boost their metabolic fitness, a keto diet can be perfect. For top athletes or those wanting to gain significant quantities of muscle or weight, it might be less desirable. The ketogenic diet is ideal in curing many diseases and reducing the risks of many diseases. There are many benefits in daily life, but it is a strict diet which requires its followers to give up eating many fruits rich in glucose. How you can follow this diet and turning it into your lifestyle is detailed discussed in this book. With more than a hundred tasty recipes, you can make your keto-friendly daily meals more delicious. Thus if you gathered up the courage to start a ketogenic diet, do not lose hope and stick to your decision as this diet is best for you.